Electroneurophysiology and Psychopathology

Advances in Biological Psychiatry

Vol. 6

Series Editors
J. Mendlewicz, Brussels and *H.M. van Praag,* Utrecht

S. Karger · Basel · München · Paris · London · New York · Sydney

2nd International Symposium on Clinical Neurophysiological Aspects of Psychopathological Conditions, Capri, September 23–26, 1980

Electroneurophysiology and Psychopathology

Volume Editors
C. Perris, Umeå, *D. Kemali* and *L. Vacca*, Naples

60 figures and 39 tables, 1981

S. Karger · Basel · München · Paris · London · New York · Sydney

Advances in Biological Psychiatry

National Library of Medicine, Cataloging in Publication
International Symposium on Clinical Neurophysiological Aspects of Psychopathological Conditions (2nd : 1980 : Capri, Italy)
Electroneurophysiology and psychopathology : 2nd International Symposium on Clinical Neurophysiological Aspects of Psychopathological Conditions, Capri, September 23–26, 1980
Volume editors, C. Perris, D. Kemali, and L. Vacca. – Basel, New York, Karger, 1981.
(Advances in biological psychiatry v. 6)
1. Electroencephalography – congresses 2. Electrophysiology – congresses 3. Mental Disorders – diagnosis – congresses 4. Neurophysiology – congresses 5. Psychopathology – congresses I. Kemali, D. II. Perris, Carlo III. Vacca, L. IV. Title V. Series
W1 AD44 v.6/[WL 102 I6592 1980e]
ISBN 3-8055-2420-X

Drug Dosage

The authors and the publisher have exerted every effort to ensure that drug selection and dosage set forth in this text are in accord with current recommendations and practice at the time of publication. However, in view of ongoing research, changes in government regulations, and the constant flow of information relating to drug therapy and drug reactions, the reader is urged to check the package insert for each drug for any change in indications and dosage and for added warnings and precautions. This is particularly important when the recommended agent is a new and/or infrequently employed drug.

Printed in Switzerland by Thür AG, Offsetdruck, Pratteln
ISBN 3-8055-2420-X

Contents

CEEG Characteristics in Relation to Vigilance, Behavioral and Cognitive Disorders, Treatment

Evoked Responses in Relation to Psychiatric Diagnoses

Acknowledgement

The publication of these proceedings has been sponsered by Lepetit SpA Milan.

List of Participants

Amati, A., Naples (Italy)
Andreoli, V., Verone (Italy)
Bartholini, G., Paris (France)
Bechtereva, N., Leningrad (USSR)
Bracale, M., Naples (Italy)
Buchsbaum, M.S., Bethesda, Md. (USA)
Campajola, P., Naples (Italy)
Connolly, T.F., London (England)
Cohen, R., Konstanz (FRG)
Cumberbatch, J., Umeå (Sweden)
Cuomo, G., Naples (Italy)
Da Prada, M., Basel (Switzerland)
Del Vecchio, M., Naples (Italy)
Di Chiara, Cagliari (Italy)
Dubini, A., Milan (Italy)
Etevenon, P., Paris (France)
Ferrari, E., Bari (Italy)
Fink, M., Stony Brook, N.Y. (USA)
Flor-Henri, P., Edmonton, Alta. (Canada)
Gaillard, J.M., Geneva (Switzerland)
Goldstein, L., Piscataway, N.J. (USA)
Grigorieva, E.A., Jaroslav (USSR)
Gruzelier, J., London (England)
Gustafson, L., Lund (Sweden)
Haefely, W., Basel (Switzerland)
Iorio, G. Naples (Italy)
Kemali, D., Naples (Italy)
Kemali, M., Naples (Italy)
Koukkou, M., Zürich (Switzerland)
Kupfer, D.J., Pittsburgh, Pa. (USA)
Longo, V.M., Naples (Italy)
Magurno, F., Naples (Italy)
Maj, M., Naples (Italy)
Marcioano, F., Naples (Italy)
Marino, A., Naples (Italy)
Matousek, M., Gothenburg (Sweden)
Mendlewicz, J., Brussels (Belgium)
Monakhov, K., Moscow (USSR)
Morocutti, C., Rome (Italy)
Muscettola, G., Naples (Italy)
Nolfe, G., Naples (Italy)
Perris, C., Umeå (Sweden)
Pinelli, P. Pavia (Italy)
Polani, P.E., London (England)
Polani, N., London (England)
Paolozzi, C., Naples (Italy)
Richter, D., Tadworth (England)
Rinaldi, F., Naples (Italy)
Saletu, B., Wien (Austria)
Shagass, C., Philadelphia, Pa. (USA)
Struwe, G., Stockholm (Sweden)
Sulg, I., Stockholm (Sweden)
Scarone, S., Milan (Italy)
Silfverskiold, P., Lund (Sweden)
Simone, F., Naples (Italy)
Timsit-Berthier, M., Liege (Belgium)
Tissot, R., Geneva (Switzerland)
Tucker, M., Grand Fork, N.Dak. (USA)
Vacca, L., Naples (Italy)
Vizioli, R., Naples (Italy)
Volvavka, J., New York, N.Y. (USA)
von Knorring, L., Umeå (Sweden)

Adv. biol. Psychiat., vol. 6, pp. 1–4 (Karger, Basel 1981)

Introduction

Electrical Neurophysiology and Psychiatry: A Look at the Past and at the Future

C. Perris, Umeå, Sweden

It is a great honour and pleasure for me to open this second international symposium on 'Neurophysiological Aspects of Psychopathological Conditions' and in such a wonderful surroundings. Prof. *Kemali* and his co-workers here in Naples are to be congratulated not only for gathering together so many distinguished colleagues, but also for giving us the opportunity to experience the splendours of this island.

The willingness with which you all accepted the invitation to participate in this symposium, which for many of you entailed a very long journey, testifies to the fact that interest in this field of research is really strong and alive. The response to the invitations has been such that the organizers' only regret is that it has proved impossible to accommodate all those research workers who would have liked to participate. I am particularly pleased with your participation because the organization of this second symposium represented a kind of reliability testing of the first one that was held in Umeå last year. Had the meeting in Umeå been a failure, you would not have been here today.

In one sense, it is symbolic that this symposium is being held on an island. When I attempted in Umeå to present a very short historical sketch of the relationship between clinical neurophysiology and psychiatry I was keen to stress that achievements in the application of clinical-neurophysiological technology to the study of psychiatric problems was made possible only because a handful research workers had believed in the relevance of this approach and had pursued it through a whole lifetime devoted to research. As you may remember, I pointed out that both clinical neurophysiologists and clinical psychiatrists very soon turned their attention away from clinical neurophysiological studies of the very complex phenomena which characterize a deranged mind toward other fields of research which appeared to them to be more rewarding in the short run. Admittedly, progress in the borderland of clinical neurophysiology and of psychiatry has been slow, and there have been more disappointments than rewards, more failures than successes. There are several reasons for this, many of them completely rational.

Firstly there is the fact that both the electrical activity of the brain, which we are able to record and analyse, and the clinical expressions of a disturbed mind, which we can observe, are dynamic processes which exhibit a very pronounced variability whithin short time limits. The situation is complicated, moreover, by the fact that we will never be able to know exactly what is going on in the mind of a fellow human being at a given moment and therefore we have to infer such psychic processes from verbal reports or behavioural cues.

Another source of error, closely related to that just mentioned, has been an over-simplicistic approach to neurophysiological studies of psychopathological manifestations both on the part of clinical neurophysiologists and on that of psychiatrists working in the field. Looking back for example at the history of EEG and psychiatry, it is now evident that important issues were improperly understood, and consequently neglected for a long time.

In EEG, one of the original approaches was mostly localizationistic and was aimed at seeking causes whereas it took a long time before it was fully realized that the EEG, as we are able to record it, is a very complex and as yet not completely understood result of processes which can easily be influenced and modified by hundreds of both internal and external factors.

Now we are more prepared to be humble and to admit that despite major progress in technical standardization, and in the standardization of the external conditions of recording, very large variations are likely to occur between the recording of one subject and that of another and also within the recording from one and the same subject on different test occasions. Moreover, the more we map the different factors which can influence the electroencephalographic end-product, the more we have to acknowledge the number of problems related to a correct interpretation of this product. If we consider, for example, that such relatively understandable variables as 'attention', 'mental ideation', and 'vigilance' can greatly influence elementary characteristics of the EEG, then we will realize that we have to cope with a kind of paradox: that is that the more we divert our attention from coarse EEG variables and focus it upon more elementary characteristics of the EEG, the more our difficulties will probably increase since these very elementary variables are likely to be influenced by different and probably uncontrollable factors.

Psychiatrists have obviously contributed to the illusion that EEG studies would help in elucidating the causes of mental disorders. Even after ideas concerning the occurrence of as yet undetected lesions lying behind most psychopathological conditions faded out and functionalistic theories were more accepted there was a strong tendency (which unfortunately still predominates in many quarters) to regard mental disorders as if they were divisible into clear-cut nosological entities with specific underlying factors proper to each one and to the whole diagnostic entity. I am sure that many of you, especially among our older colleagues, will easily remember the hypothesis of a similarity in the neurophysiological mechanisms underlying epilepsy and schizophrenia which was generated in the 1940s and 1950s by a misunderstanding on the part of psychiatrists of the occurrence of schizophrenia-like psychoses of an epileptic origin and by the proneness in psychiatric quarters to regard schizophrenia as a unitary disease.

I understand that it was an increased awareness of the width of all these problems which led many of our colleages – some of whom are present here today – to direct their efforts towards studies of the dynamic aspects of brain neurophysiology, for example studies of the reactivity of the brain to external stimuli.

Studies of EEG characteristics where a time component was taken into account and studies of reactivity to external stimuli have yielded important results, which I do not need to review at this juncture since many of them will emerge from your own contributions to this meeting. However, one of the major obstacles to a closer understanding of these findings still remained: namely the inadequacy of the current diagnostic concepts. In fact, the evolution towards a standardization of diagnostic procedures, and the understanding that clinical syndromes held together by a common label might in reality be comprised of quite different elements with different underlying mechanisms has occurred much more slowly than the standardization of clinical neurophysiological methods for collecting data and analysing them.

In a previous paper [*Perris* et al., 1978] we have stressed that psychiatric diagnostic classifications can only be regarded as a rough basis for delimiting the field of investigation. We have also pointed out that clinical diagnoses cannot be regarded as an appropriate clinical measure for comparison with measures of the elementary characteristics of neurophysiological brain activity (or reactivity) which we are now able to obtain since these variables refer to different levels of integration. Furthermore, since it was perfectly clear to us that our neurophysiological measures refer to time-bound events, we have stressed that much more care than before should be taken to obtain for our comparisons, clinical variables which are as closely related as possible in time to the neurophysiological ones which are measured. I will not dwell on this at this juncture, since I myself still feel somewhat uncomfortable about my own position on the issue of whether we should look at the possible relationships between clinical and neurophysiological events within an epiphenomenalistic frame of reference, or whether we should consider those relationships as an expression of phenomena occurring concomitantly at different levels without making, for the time being, any inference about cause and effect. I hope, however, that the work of this symposium will also contribute to the further clarification of this important issue.

I would like to return for a while to my symbolic image of our work occurring on an island, or at least in some sort of frontier land. It seems to me, in fact, that we who work with neurophysiological aspects of psychiatry are looked upon with a certain amount of scepticism by both neurophysiologists and psychiatrists.

The former, who have increasingly concentrated their studies to single elements of the nervous system, often carried out under well standardized laboratory conditions, cannot quite understand how we can continue to rely on methods which give us results that are difficult to interpret and which are loaded with several sources of error. The psychiatrists also look at us askance because our results so far are not suitable for more immediate practical application, or because our approach to the study of mental disorders is not quite in line with more fashionable psychiatric conceptions. We are working in the frontier country between scientific idealism and clinical pragmatism and I suspect that we will remain there for some time to come.

During the last few years, however, a fair number of results have been accumulating which show a reasonable level of consistency both across different laboratories, and across different techniques of analysis. At the same time, progress has occurred in the ascertainment and in the measurement of more closely defined psychopathological variables, which has contributed to the establishment of a narrower, but also more suitable basis for the search for possible relationships between clinical and neurophysiological events. To these achievements, which in themselves cannot be overlooked, must be added on the one hand an increasing body of knowledge concerning the close relationship between neurophysiological measures and biochemical variables, and on the other hand the repeated documentation of a possible specific influence that different psychotropic drugs exert upon neurophysiological events. Taking all this progress into account, I feel more comfortable as regards neurophysiological studies of psychopathological conditions and of their treatment and more optimistic about the possible future rewards for our efforts.

Finally, I believe strongly that meetings like this one, which allow people with a specific and thorough training in either neurophysiological techniques or psychopathological assessment or in both to get together and share their experiences provide one of the best forums not only because they encourage self-criticism but also because they enable us to co-ordinate our efforts towards the achievement of future goals.

Reference

Perris, C.; Monakhov, K.; Knorring, L. von; Botskarev, V.; Nikiforov, A.: Systemic structural analysis of the electroencephalogram of depressed patients. General principles and preliminary results of an international collaborative study. Neuropsychobiology *4:* 207–228 (1978).

C. Perris, MD, Department of Psychiatry, University of Umeå,
S-901 85 Umeå (Sweden)

Adv. biol. Psychiat., vol. 6, pp. 5–11 (Karger, Basel 1981)

A Reflection of Physiological Mechanism or a Programme of Brain Activity

K. Monakhov

Instute of Psychiatry, Academy of Medical Science, Moscow, USSR

For this communication we used data which were obtained in our collaborative Soviet-Swedish programme and results accumulated in our laboratory in Moscow in previous years. The results were obtained both by studying normals and patients with schizophrenia and depressive syndromes of different aetiology. The idea which will be discussed now was formulated in connection with the main problem of clinical EEG in psychiatry: the possibility of a reflection of the mental processes and their pathology in electrical brain activity.

If we trace a history of the problem the following sequence of methodological approaches will be obtained. In the early time of development of EEG technique neurophysiologists rested their hopes on the idea that a detailed analysis of brain waves would give information about mental processes. But this was not realized. The next step was that mental processes could be reflected in reactive changes of electrical activity depending upon different kinds of stimuli.

Many attempts were made using combinations of psychological tasks and registration of EEG. But the problem is how to analyse electrical activity adequately for comparing it with physiological data.

In the last two decades, thanks to computer techniques, investigators again tried to find out some reflection of specific brain processes in electrical characteristics. Very shortly this approach can be classified as follows. Some of the computer analyses are directed to describe characteristics of EEG, such as amplitude, frequency, shapes of the waves and so on. There are two possibilities for this: to use Fourier analysis and some other formal mathematical analysis or to use techniques of automatized visual-manual routine clinical EEG analysis [15]. After this step one builds up histogrames of characteristics to compare results of different clinical states. In some investigations neurophysiologists go further and apply factorial, discriminant analysis, a techinque of conjunctive combination and so on to describe electrical brain activity as a system [5, 11].

The results obtained in our laboratory enable us to state now that EEG does not give sufficient information about physiological mechanisms nor mental activity.

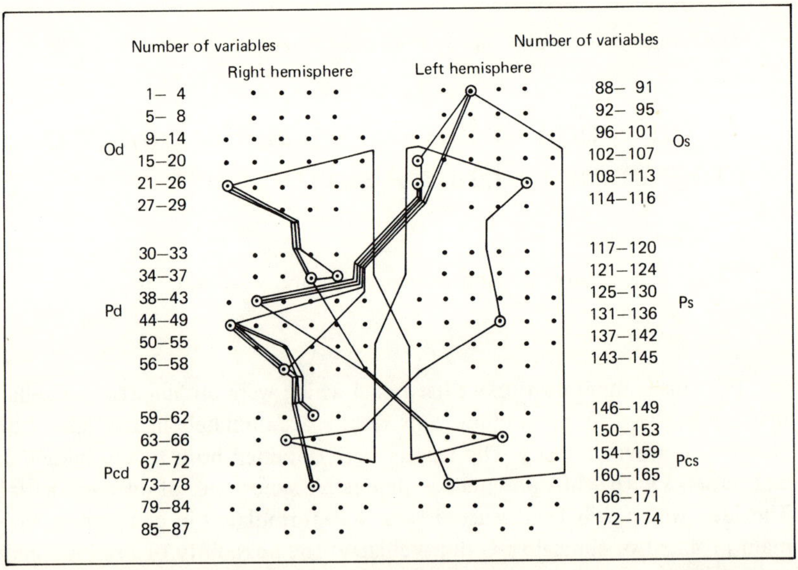

Fig. 1. Neurofunctional systems in depressive syndrome. On the left and right margins – numbers of EEG characteristics. Lines between characteristics indicate combinations of them. Od = occipital region, right; Pd = pazietal region, right; Pcd = precentral, right; Os = occipital region, left; Ps = pazietal region, left; Pcs = precentral, left.

There are many samples where the EEG in different behavioural and mental conditions shows only variations of the amplitude-frequency spectrum which testify to some changes in electrical activity in structures but which are not specific for these conditions.

We guess that the weak information of EEG in relation to mechanisms of behavioural reactions of men and animals is based upon two theses. Firstly, genesis of the general electrical activity is stipulated for many factors. It depends on both synaptic [3, 4], dendritic [6, 18] glial processes [19], and on circulatory and metabolic processes [1]. All this exists in a volume conductor of a complex nature with active capacities and resistors, with oriented dipoles. That is why it is very difficult to speak about a neurophysiological mechanism or even more about functional states of structures. Secondly, if one even accepts the possibility of the reflection of physiological processes in electrical processes, the modern point of view on physiological mechanisms of behaviour is based upon the idea that this mechanism includes coordinated activity of a lot of morphological-functional structures provided by means of their systemic organization [2, 7–10, 12, 20]. Consequently, an investigation of single structures can give only a part of physiological mechanism separated from the whole mechanism. Naturally,

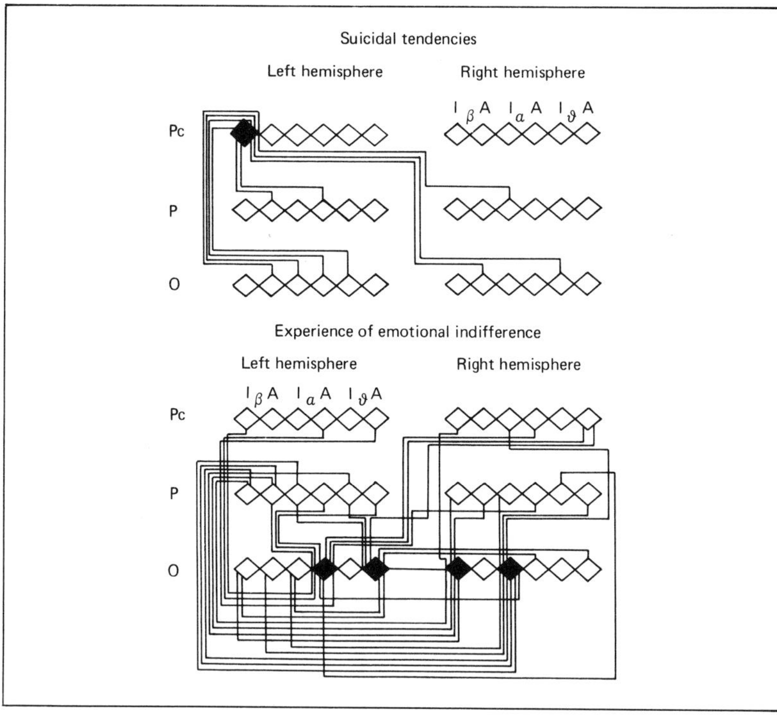

Fig. 2. Neurofunctional systems in depressive symptoms. Each rhombus = index or amplitude of beta, alpha and theta waves of EEG. Lines between them indicate combinations of different EEG characteristics in brain areas. Pc = precentral region; P = parietal region; O = occipital region.

this cannot give sufficient information about neurophysiological mechanisms of behaviour and mental activity.

Several years ago we proposed the concept of functional stratification in brain processes and conforming systemic-structural analysis [12]. *Perris* and myself together with our collaborators [13, 14, 16, 17] conducted investigations of electrical activity in normals and patients with depressive syndromes on the basis of this concept. As a result of the investigations it was possible to describe a so-called bioelectrical structure (BES) and neurofunctional system (NFS). The BES consists of interconnected primary characteristics of different brain area EEGs. The NFS represents a system of the BES which is regularly revealed in EEGs of a certain mental state (or syndrome) or purposeful behaviour. As a sample, the NFS in depressive syndrome is shown in figure 1.

This kind of NFS was determined in EEG of schizophrenic patients with continuous and periodical forms [9], in the EEG of depressed patients of different aetiology [16] and in relation to individual symptoms of depression (fig. 2) [14, 17]. In all these cases NFSs have sufficient correlation with the clinical characteristics enough to use them for automatic classification of this psychopathology (table I). A similar investigation was performed in the course of trace-conditioned reflex elaboration in healthy subjects and schizophrenics with a defective state (fig. 3) [10].

All this, we think, testifies to the correlation of systemic characteristics of the electrical activity with behavioural and mental processes. But every neurophysiological investigation requires an interpretation of a physiological mechanism of those states or activities which were investigated. This difficult problem was in our mind for a long time and now it is possible to formulate a consideration as follows. As our results indicate, it is possible to give only a general interpretation about physiological mechanisms of brain activity. A description of the mechanism was given in terms of Pavlov physiology, in terms of excitation and inhibition and their spatial distribution. Until now we could not give any more details of the analysis. For understanding the matter of a disease this, naturally, is not enough. But even this interpretation is based upon a hypothetical notion about fast activity as an index of excitation and slow activity as an index of inhibition in corresponding brain structures.

The reasons make us return to the question: What reflects general electrical activity? It is evident that NFS is related to psychopathological states inasmuch as the characteristics of NFS regularly correlate with clinical characteristics. But this correlation is not based on physiological mechanisms, it is based on spatial-temporary organization of functional parts of unknown physiological mechanisms.

To clarify this idea I shall draw an analogy. If we have a complex apparatus, two aspects of its function can be investigated: the aspect of the interaction of its functioning parts or blocks and the aspect of its mechanism of function. For the first aspect it is enough to use some external indices of its function, such as temperature, noise, electrical potentials, and so on, and a description of their interconnections. Such a description will be sufficient for a descrimination of this apparatus from another or to characterize its 'behaviour' in different conditions. For the second aspect – understanding of the mechanism – we must study each block, explain its specific function and its connections with the other blocks existing in the whole apparatus. After this it is possible to give a complete description of its principle organization and purpose.

Thus, neurophysiologists who deal with psychiatry are faced with two aims: to give a description of a purpose of each part of a physiological mechanism and describe a type of their organization in the whole physiological system. We call this second aspect a neurofunctional programme of the brain activity.

According to the analogy mentioned above, we can describe a type of functional organization using external indices of the brain activity without knowl-

Table I. Computer classification between continuous and periodical forms of schizophrenia (experimental groups) and between control groups[1]

	Experimental groups	Control groups
Number of combinations	45	5
Percentage of correct classification	83	25
Percentage of uncertainty	13	75
Percentage of mistaken classification	4	0

[1] Two groups containing equal portions of continuous and periodical forms of schizophrenia in each.

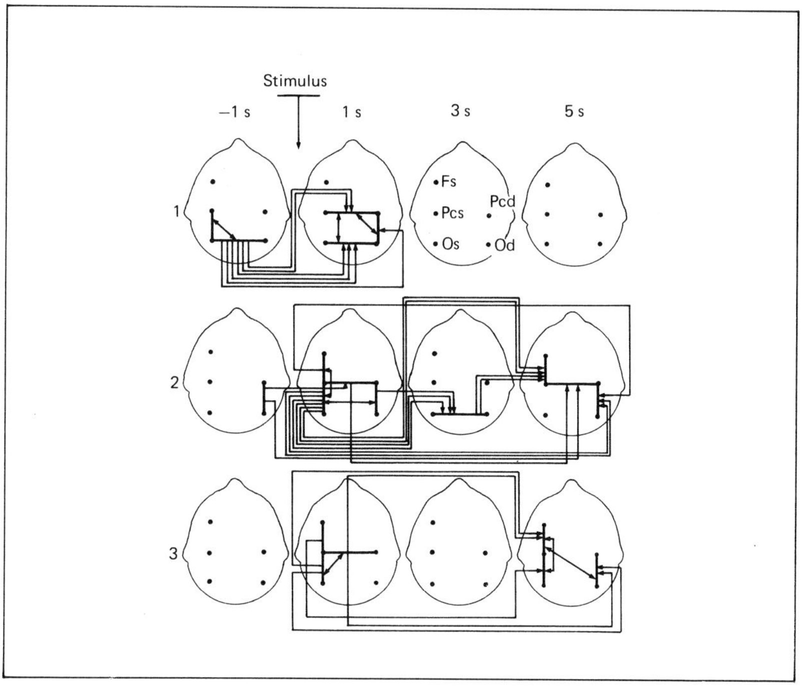

Fig. 3. Neurofunctional systems in the course of trace motor conditioned reflex elaboration (5 s delayed). Thick lines between points = correlation coeffitients of evoked activity in corresponding areas; thin lines with arrows = combinations between correspondent coefficients. 1 = NFS with different stimuli; 2 = NFS with stable trace-conditioned reflex in healthy subjects; 3 = NFS with non-elaborated reflex in schizophrenic patients in a defect state. Fs = frontal region, left; Pcs = precentral, left; Os = occipital, left; Pcd = precentral region, right; Od = occipital, right.

edge of its mechanism and based only on regular correlation of these indices with specific functions of the brain. EEG gives us this opportunity.

The understanding of the EEG's role as an index of the neurofunctional programme in the investigation of brain activity allows us to adequately determine possibilities and limitations of the EEG method and its more effective application.

The study and the description of neurofunctional programmes in different diseases, and psychopathological states, in the studies of the efficacy of psychopharmacological drugs, enable us to make a significant contribution to clinical psychiatry. The features of neurofunctional programmes in various psychopathological states allow us to elaborate a more adequate classification – a clinico-neurophysiological classification. Well known are the works with EEG application aimed at determination of psychotropic properties of drugs, as well as at that of their efficacy prediction [5]. All this is done on the basis of the programme aspect studies of brain activity without sufficient knowledge of the internal physiological mechanisms of the disease or a particular state.

Summary

On the basis of a systemic structural analysis, so-called bioelectrical structures (BES) were eleborated. They represent a system of interconnection between characteristics of the brain electrical activity in different functional areas. A neurofunctional system which consists of interconnected BES rather reflects a programme of functional organization of the brain than neurophysiological mechanisms. The peculiarities of these programmes in different mental and behavioural conditions permit one to use them for understanding brain activity and for classifying different clinical states.

References

1 Aladzalova, N.A.: Slow electrical processes in the brain (in Russian) (Nauka, Moscow 1962).

2 Anokhin, P.K.: Essays on physiology of functional systems (in Russian) (Medicina, Moscow 1975).

3 Frost, J.D.; Gol, A.: Computer determination of relationships between EEG activity and single unit descharges in isolated cortex. Expl. Neurol. *14:* 506 (1966).

4 Jasper, H.H.; Stefanis, C.: Intracellular ascillatory rhythms in pyramidal cells of cat. Electroenceph. clin. Neurophysiol. *18:* 541 (1965).

5 Itil, T.M.: Quantitative pharmaco-EEG in the discovery of psychotropic properties of drugs; in Neuro-psychopharmacology, pp. 1183–1190 (Pergamon Press, Oxford, 1978).

6 Klee, M.R.; Offenloch, K.; Tigges, J.: Cross-correlation analysis of electroencephalographic potentials and membran transiens. Science *147:* 519 (1965).

7 Livanov, M.N.: Spatial organization of the brain processes (in Russian) (Nauka, Moscow 1972).

8 Monakhov, K.K.: The Pavlovian theory in psychiatry: some recent developments; in

Modern perspectives in world psychiatry, No. 2, pp. 531–556 (Oliver & Boyd, Edinburgh 1968).

9 Monakhov, K.K.; Epstein, G.; Lobacheva, V.; Botskarev, V.; Leibovitsh, F.; Sundukova, Z.; Nikiforov, A.: Application of computer differetial diagnostic method for investigation of systemic brain activity (in Russian). Zh. Nevropat. Psychiat. *72:* 481–486 (1972).

10 Monakhov, K.K.; Rumjantseva, L.K.; Lobacheva, V.P.: Spatial-temporal system of connections of evoked activity in human conditioned reactions (in Russian). Zh. vyssh. nerv. Deyat. I.P. Pavlova *23:* 366–374 (1973).

11 Monakhov, K.; Epstein, G.; Nikiforov, A.; Botskarev, V.: Formal mathematical methods for the investigation of relationships between electrical activity of the brain and mental phenomena (in Russian). Zh. vyssh. nerv. Deyat. I.P. Pavlova *24:* 202–208 (1974).

12 Monakhov, K.K.: Concept of functional stratification of mental and higher nervous activity (in Russian). Zh. vyssh. nerv. Deyat. I.P. Pavlova *26:* 4–7 (1976).

13 Monakhov, K.K.; Perris, C.; Botskarev, V.; Knorring, L. von; Nikiforov, A.: Functional interhemispheric differences in relation to various psychopathological components of depressive syndromes. Neuropsychobiology *5:* 143–155 (1979).

14 Monakhov, K.K.; Perris, C.: Neurophysiological correlates of depressive symptomatology *6:* 268–279 (1980).

15 Nikiforov, A.I.; Botskarev, V.K.: Primary analysis of human EEG by means of small digital computers (in Russian). Zh. Nevropat. Psykhiat. *74:* 288–292 (1974).

16 Perris, C.; Monakhov, K.; Knorring, L. von; Botskarev, V.; Nikiforov, A.: Systemic structural analysis of the EEG of depressed patients. Neuropsychobiology *4:* 207–228 (1978).

17 Perris, C.; Monakhov, K.: Depressive symptomatology and systemic structural analysis of the EEG; in Gruzelier, Flor-Henry, Hemisphere asymmetries of function in psychopathology, pp. 223–236 (Elsevier, Amsterdam 1979).

18 Purpura, D.P.: Nature of electrocortical potentials and synaptic organizations in cerebral and cerebellar cortex. Int. Rev. Neurobiol. *1:* 47–163 (1959).

19 Roitbak, A.I.: Slow cortical negative potentials and neuroglia; in Modern problems in physiology and pathology of the nervous system (in Russian), p. 68 (Moscow 1965).

20 Shvirkov, V.B.: Neurophysiological investigations of systemic mechanism of behaviour (in Russian) (Nauka, Moscow 1978).

Prof. K.K. Monakhov, Institute of Psychiatry, Academy of Medical Science,
Zogorodnoje Sh. 2, Bld. 2, 113152 Moscow (USSR)

Adv. biol. Psychiat., vol. 6, pp. 12–16 (Karger, Basel 1981)

Statistical Organizational Features of the Computerized EEG under Various Behavioral States

Leonide Goldstein[1]

CMDNJ-Rutgers Medical School, Piscataway, N.J., USA

The hypothesis that certain cortical functional states are detectible in features of the statistical organization of the quantitated EEG was first formulated by *Liberson* [1936], *Chweitzer* et al. [1936] and *Drohocki* [1937] who pointed out that in normal human subjects, in a state of sustained arousal, the distributions of repeated successive measurements of the amplitudes around their means were most often Gaussian. These distributions changed in a characteristic way according to certain behavioral states and under drug-induced mental abnormalities.

These findings were confirmed in studies performed on hallucinating chronic schizophrenics and normal subjects treated with LSD-25 [*Goldstein* et al., 1963, 1965]. In both cases, the scatter of measurement values around their respective means was, in the left occipital, one half that present in normal controls.

With the extension of quantitated EEG studies to both right (R) and left (L) sides of the brain, hemispheric differences for certain behavioral features were found. *D'Elia and Perris* [1973] reported that in untreated depressed patients the variance of the distribution of EEG amplitudes was twice or more higher in the R than in the L, a difference which disappeared following effective treatment. *Goldstein* [1975] found a similar, although less pronounced, difference between academically successful and unsuccessful students. This feature was confirmed in a study on a large number of subjects [*Wiet and Goldstein,* 1979].

The present paper extends this type of EEG analysis to other groups of subjects with particular behavioral characteristics and to mental patients with depression and acute schizophrenia.

[1] I express my gratitude to *Charmion Semple, Philip Oltman, Robert Karlin,* and *Steve Wiet* for the permission to use unpublished data obtained in collaborative studies.

Methods

The EEG recordings were obtained with gold-plated cup electrodes from T4-T3, with Cz as common reference and the middle forehead for grounding, on a Beckman type RM polygraph, filtering out the frequencies below 0.5 and above 30 Hz. (Other leads were used but the data obtained will not be mentioned in this paper.) Analog-integrators were used to perform on-line amplitude measurements, without separation according to the conventional frequency bands.

The numerical values of the amplitudes cumulated over successive epochs of 5-sec duration (40–60 artefact-free) were processed off-line to obtain the statistical parameters to be presented. The computer program performed a classification of the individual measurements within 10 equal classes, the values of which were derived from the arithmetic difference between the lowest and highest value encountered. This yielded frequency distribution histograms. Next, a probit transformation was performed [*Bliss,* 1935; *Fisher and Yates,* 1957]. The number of modes of each individual histogram was determined from the number of regression lines needed to obtain the least-square residuals.

All sessions took place in a sound- and light-attenuated room, with the subjects in the reclining position. The procedures were carefully described and consent was obtained. For the normal subjects a small financial reward was provided. Except in the case of field-dependent-independent subjects, the recordings were performed in the eye-closed condition.

Results

1. Mental Patients

The results obtained on 38 inpatients (20 with a diagnosis of neurotic depression and 18 with a diagnosis of acute paranoid schizophrenia) are listed in table I. For comparative purpose 20 normal subjects are included, even though their age range is smaller than that of the patients.

As can be seen, in normals there was no difference between the mean number of modes in the distributions of R and L amplitudes. In untreated depressed patients, the number of modes was 1.6 times higher in the R than in the L temporal leads, a highly significant statistical difference. At discharge (3–4 weeks after admission, as a result of treatment with tricyclic antidepressants) from recordings obtained on half of the patients (the other half having refused to submit to the procedure, or having left before it could be implemented) it can be seen that there was a near equalization of the number of modes between the hemispheres. It should be noted, however, that at that point the actual values were significantly higher than those found in normal volunteers.

In the case of schizophrenic patients, a reversal of the relations existing in depressed patients was found, since the number of modes in the L was 1.5 times higher than in the R: this was also a statistically significant difference. Also, as the patients improved as a result of treatment with neuroleptics, an equalization of the modes occurred. Contrary to the depressed patients, at discharge the mean number of modes was not different from that of the normals. In none of the three groups was there a significant difference between males and females.

Table I. Mean number of modes (±SE) in the distribution of EEG amplitudes. Temporal leads, eyes closed

					At admission			At discharge	
Diagnosis	N	M	F	Age range	right	left	n	right	left
Normals	20	11	9	18–22	1.85 ± 0.18*	1.90 ± 0.18*	–	–	–
Depression	20	6	14	18–55	4.05 ± 0.29	2.55 ± 0.25**	9	3.22 ± 0.28	3.11 ± 0.31
Schizophrenia	18	11	7	18–64	2.44 ± 0.28	3.55 ± 0.22**	15	2.40 ± 0.21	2.73 ± 0.23

* Statistically significant difference for both R and L with both groups of patients (t-test, $p<0.05$).
** Statistically significant difference between R and L (t-test $p<0.05$).

Table II. Mean number of modes (±SE) in the right + left distributions of amplitudes in field-dependent male subjects. Data from *Semple, Oltman and Goldstein,* unpublished

Condition	Field-independent (n=8)	Field-dependent (n = 8)
Eyes closed	1.69 ± 0.34	1.37 ± 0.20
Eyes opened	1.50 ± 0.13	2.19 ± 0.19*

* Statistically significant difference (paired t-test = 2.99 $p<0.01$).

Table III. Mean number of modes (± SE) in the distribution of amplitudes in low, moderate and high-hypnotizable subjects. Temporal leads, pre-hypnosis baseline, eyes closed

Hypnotic susceptibility	N	Mean number of modes
Low	10	1.45 ± 0.15
Moderate	17	2.05 ± 0.18*
High	21	2.61 ± 0,18**

* Statistically significant difference one-tailed t-test: $p < 0.05$.
** Statistically significant difference one-tailed t-test: $p = 0.05$.

2. *Behavioral Characteristics*

16 carefully selected male subjects [rod and frame and embedded figure tests, *Witkin,* 1971], of which 8 were at the extreme of field dependence (FD) and 8 at the extreme of field independence (FI) were recorded under eye-closed and eye-open conditions following each other without interruption. The results are presented in table II.

In that series of experiments, as in the one to be presented next, there was no significant difference between the number of modes in the R and L hemispheres. Therefore, the data presented reflect the global R + L/2 number of modes, for each subject, under each condition.

As can be seen, in FI there was no change in the mean number of modes between the two conditions. In FD subjects the mean number of modes was slightly lower than in FI subjects under the eye-closed situation, but the difference was not significant. However, there was in the FD subjects a marked, highly significant increase in the mean number of modes when they shifted from the eye-closed to the eye-open condition.

In the case of hypnotizability studies, recordings were performed on three groups selected on the basis of the Stanford Hypnotic Susceptibility Scale Form C [*Weitzenhoffer and Hilgard,* 1967]. The mean number of modes across hemispheres was found to be linearly related to the degree of hypnotizability (table III).

Discussion

The common denominator of these different studies is an attempt to relate EEG-based appraisal of cortical functional states to behavioral states or characteristics. Although still limited in scope as well as in the number of individual subjects recorded from, it does seem that such a relation exists.

In the matter of psychopathology there have been numerous studies, using a variety of measurement methods implicating the L hemisphere in schizophrenia and the R hemisphere in depression. The present investigations support these conclusions; however, the data at hand seem to indicate that rather than a L or R dysfunction, one may be dealing with a disruption of the inter-hemispheric relationships which could lead to a partial impairment of the mutual control. This is indicated by the fact that in both depression as well as schizophrenia, improvement is manifested by an equalization of the statistical organization of the electrical activity between the hemispheres.

In the case of the field dependence-independence behavioral dimension the striking fact is that a global increase in the complexity of the statistical organization occurs only in those subjects (FD) who are known to process actively the features of their surroundings. The fact that this occurs in both hemispheres at the same time may indicate that it affects both visual-spatial and verbal-analytical processes.

Finally, a somewhat similar mechanism might be involved in the phenomenon of hypnotizability. A number of authors have related hypnotic susceptibility to the capacity to focus attention [*Hilgard,* 1970]. It can be hypothesized that the more one pays attention, the more one has to process at the same time. The increase in the number of modes in the distribution of EEG amplitudes might well correspond to individual capabilities for such processes.

Summary

Statistical studies of the distribution of EEG amplitudes in the right (R) and left (L) temporals (probit analysis) were performed during successive measurements obtained at rest. There is a significantly larger number of modes in the R than in the L in untreated depressives, while in acute schizophrenics the reverse is found, i.e. significantly larger number in the L than in the R. In both types of patients equalization of the modes occurs with improvement. Differences in the number of modes have been found in field-dependent but not in field-independent subjects between eyes-closed and eyes-open conditions, and between low, moderate and high hypnotizable subjects with eyes closed.

References

Bliss, C.I.: The calculation of the dosage-mortality curve. Ann. appl. Biol. *22:* 134–167 (1935).

Chweitzer, A.; Geblewicz, E.; Liberson, W.: Action de la mescaline sur les ondes alpha (Rhythme de Berger chez l'homme). C.r. Séanc. Soc. Biol. *124:* 1296–1299 (1936).

D'Elia, G.; Perris, C.: Cerebral function dominance and depression. Acta psychiat. scand. *49:* 191–197 (1973).

Drohocki, Z.: Die spontane elektrische Spannungsproduktion der Grosshirnrinde. Pflügers Arch ges. Physiol. *239:* 658–679 (1937).

Fisher, R.A.; Yates, F.: Statistical tables for biological, agricultural and medical research (Hafner, New York 1957).

Goldstein, L.; Murphree, H.B.; Sugerman, A.A.; Pfeiffer, C.C.; Jenney, E.H.: Quantitative electroencephalographic analysis of naturally occurring (schizophrenic) and drug-induced psychotic states in human males. Clin. Pharmacol. Ther. *4:* 10–21 (1963).

Goldstein, L.; Sugerman, A.A.; Stolberg, H.; Murphree, H.B.; Pfeiffer, C.C.: Electrocerebral activity in schizophrenic and non-psychotic subjects. Quantitative EEG amplitude analysis. Electroenceph. clin. Neurophysiol. *19:* 350–361 (1965).

Goldstein, L.: Time domain analysis of the EEG. The integrative method; in Dolce, Kunkel, Cean, pp. 251–270 (Fischer, Stuttgart 1975).

Hilgard, J.R.: Personality and hypnosis: a study of imaginative involvement (University of Chicago Press, Chicago 1970).

Liberson, W.: Electroencephalographie transcranienne chez l'homme. Trav. Hum. *4:* 303–320 (1936).

Weitzenhoffer, A.; Hilgard, E.: Revised Stanford Profile Scales of Hypnotic Susceptibility (Consulting Psychologists Press, Palo Alto 1967).

Wiet, S.; Goldstein, L.: Successful and unsuccessful university students: quantitative hemispheric EEG differences. Biol. Psychol. *8:* 273–284 (1979).

Witkin, H.A.: The embedded figure test (Consulting Psychologists Press, Palo Alto 1971).

L. Goldstein, DSc, CMDNJ-Rutgers Medical School, Piscataway, NJ 08540 (USA)

Adv. biol. Psychiat., vol. 6, pp. 17–28 (Karger, Basel 1981)

CEEG Findings in Schizophrenics, Depressives, Obsessives, Heroin Addicts and Normals[1]

D. Kemali[a], *L. Vacca*[a], *F. Marciano*[b], *G. Nolfe*[b], *G. Iorio*[a],[2]

Consistent quantitative EEG deviations in patients with major psychoses have been found, but the precise nature of these abnormalities and their diagnostic specificity is still to be determined [*Abrams and Taylor,* 1979]. Several studies have shown that EEG of schizophrenics have a greater power at beta frequencies and lower in the alpha band [*Giannitrapani and Kayton,* 1974; *Itil* et al., 1974] and lateralized asymmetrical as well as inter-area dysfunctions [*Franzen and Ingvar,* 1975; *Flor-Henry* et al., 1979a, b; *Gur* 1979]. In affective psychoses and obsessive patients, *Flor-Henry* et al. [1979a, b] recently showed bitemporal and left temporal EEG differences compared with normals. *Perris* et al. [1978] and *Monakhov* et al. [1979] observed EEG deviations and interhemispheric functional differences in depressed patients. Opiate and polydrug users also showed EEG deviations mostly condensed in low frequencies [*Alberti,* 1976; *Grant and Judd,* 1976; *Judd* et al., 1978]. The present study is part of a long-term EEG research program on psychiatric patients and drug abusers that we are carrying out in order to verify our previous method and results, to compare them with those of other investigators, and in particular for schizophrenics in order to evaluate if variables other than the psychiatric disorder may interfere with the EEG quantitative deviations [*Shagass* et al., 1979].

Method and Subjects

67 schizophrenics, 22 depressives (8 unipolar endogenous, 14 neurotic reactive), 5 obsessive short-term inpatients, and 31 heroin addicts were subjected to a multichannel resting EEG record. 76 healthy volunteers, selected for number, sex and age, were sub-

[a] Clinica Psychiatrica, Prima Facoltà di Medicina-Chirurgia, Università di Napoli e [b] Istituto di Cibernetica, Sezione di Bioelettronica del CNR Arco Felice, Napoli, Italia

[1] The research was supported in part by grant CT 780214004 of CNR and in part by funds of Min. Pub. Istr. cap. 8551/1979.

[2] The authors wish to thank Mr. *D'Angelo* (Psychiatric Unit) and Mr. *Di Franco* (Institute of Cybernetics) of the CNR for their technical assistance.

grouped as controls strictly comparable to the experimental groups. The patients had been drug-free for at least 14 days prior to EEG registrations, and none had ever received convulsant therapy. All of the patients were in a clear state of consciousness and no diagnosable structural disease of the central nervous system and no medical illness known to cause psychiatric symptoms or EEG deviations had been found in the experimental groups. The drug addicts were chronic heroin users; the EEGs were recorded 7 or 8 h after the last injection of heroin and no withdrawal symptoms occurred during the registrations. For formal diagnostic categories the patients were classified according to the ICD-9 of the World Health Organization. The research diagnostic criteria required for schizophrenia were at least two of Schneider's first-rank symptoms [*Schneider,* 1966], and for depression the criteria of *Perris* [1966] were followed. For chronic schizophrenia (n = 38) the criteria according to *Feighner* et al. [1972] and *Astrachan* et al. [1972] were adopted; 29 schizophrenics were in a state of acute exacerbation. The severity of symptoms was scored according to the Comprehensive Psychopathological Rating Scale [*Asberg* et al., 1976]. For depressive patients Hamilton's Scale for Depression was also used. The subjects handedness was tested by means of the *Raczkowsky* et al. [1974] questionnaire. As for as the EEG recording procedure and computation are concerned the method is described in detail elsewhere [*Kemali* et al., 1980a; *Marciano and Nolfe,* 1980]. For the EEG spectral analysis the following descriptors were used: the relative activity (RA), the barycentric frequency (BF) and the barycentric radius (BR). All the data were statistically evaluated as follows: the Student t test and the Mann-Whitney test for intergroup comparisons, and the correlate t test and the Wilcoxon test for the interhemispheric confrontations. Only those data that were in the probability of $p \leqslant 0.05$ for both tests employed respectively in the intergroup and interhemispheric comparisons were considered significant. The Kolmogorov-Smirnof test was used for evaluating the function of distribution. Serum prolactin levels were calculated by the method of *Hwang* et al. [1971] in 52 schizophrenics, 21 depressives, 4 obsessives, 31 heroin addicts and 43 healthy controls.

Results

Compared with healthy controls the schizophrenics showed a significantly higher beta BF and BR in both frontal and parietal leads. The beta BR was higher in the occipital areas too. In the group of schizophrenics the frontal and parietal alpha RA was lower and the delta RA was higher. The schizophrenics also had higher beta RA in all leads explored, but the values were not significant for all the statistical tests employed (fig. 1). The depressives, when compared with healthy controls, showed lower delta BR in parietal, occipital areas and in the right frontal area.

The alpha BR was higher in the left frontal and parietal as well as in the right occipital channel (fig. 2). The differences between the small sample of obsessives and healthy controls were highly different in the first and second comparisons (fig. 3), then they have not been considered as consistent data. Heroin addicts had a higher theta RA than controls in parietal and occipital leads as well as in the left frontal lead (fig. 4). As shown in table I, chronic schizophrenics had a higher frontal and parietal theta. BF than schizophrenics suffering from epi-

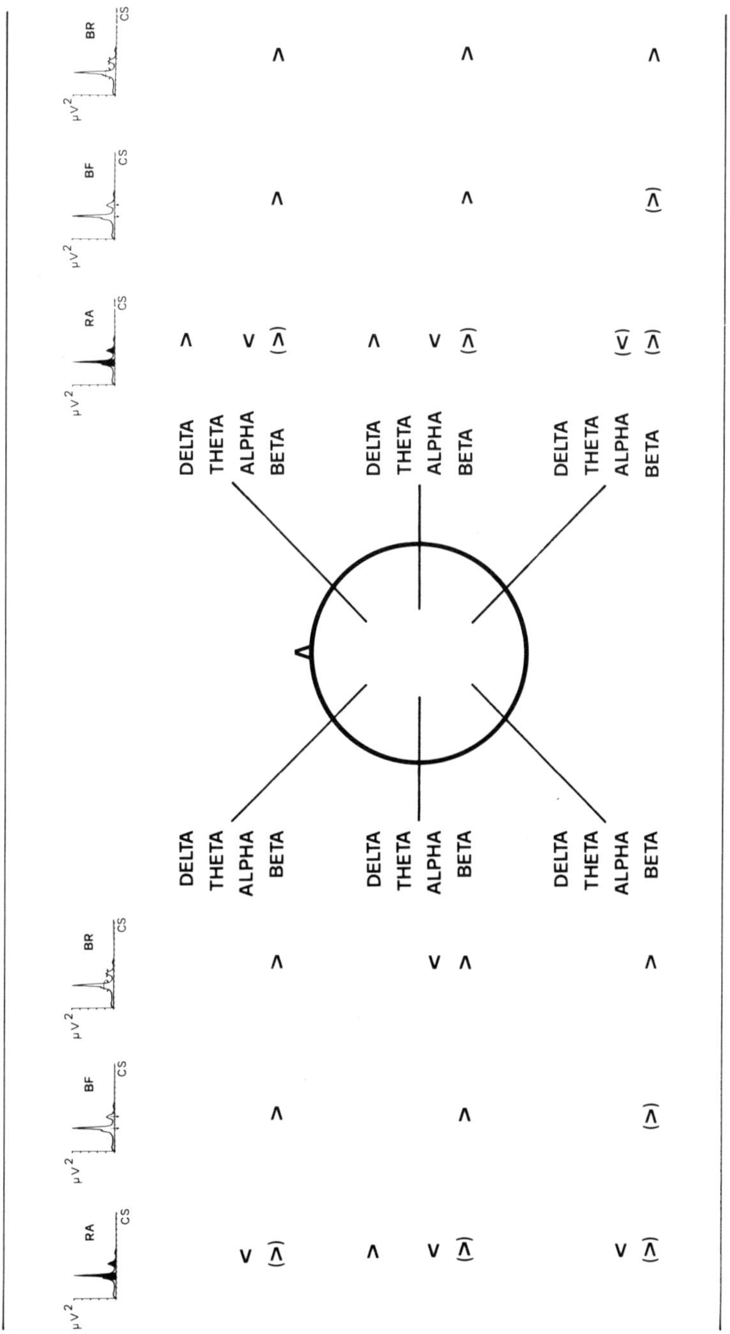

Fig. 1. Schizophrenics (n = 67) *(A)* versus controls (n = 65) *(B)*. > indicates higher and < lower values in the first group; when in parentheses, (>) and (<) denote values exceeding the level of significance in one of the statistical tests employed ($p \leqslant 0.05$).

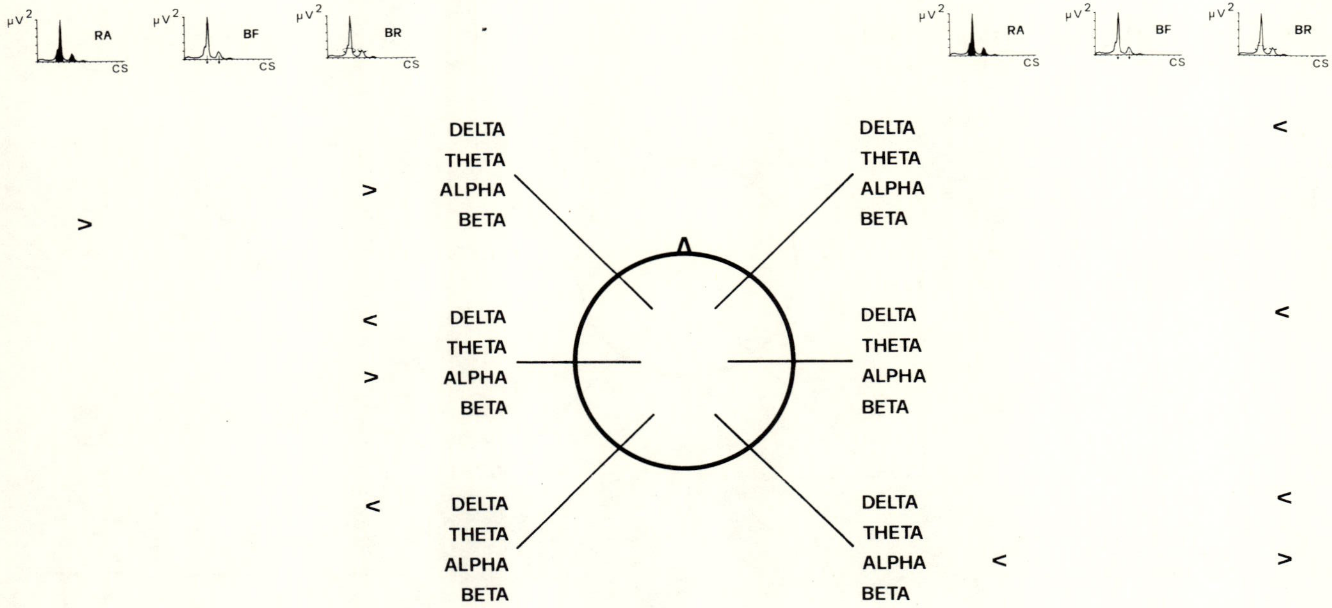

Fig. 2. Depressives (n = 22) *(A)* versus controls (n = 22 *(B)*. > indicates higher and < lower values in the first group ($p \leqslant 0.05$).

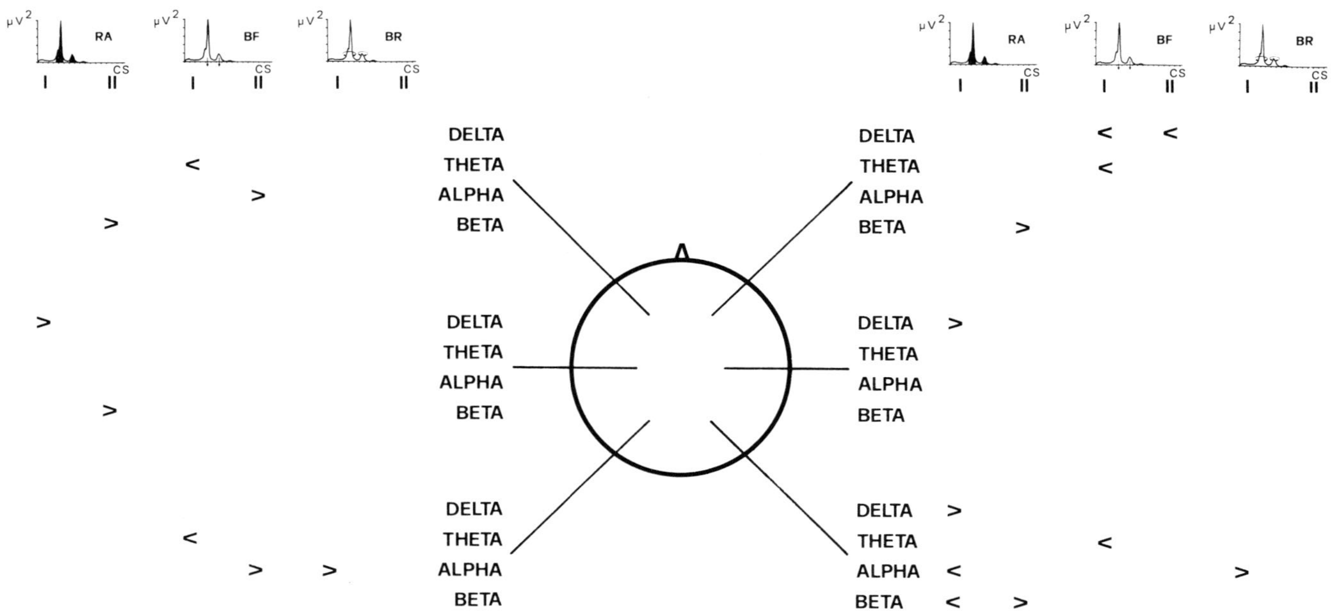

Fig. 3. Obsessives (n = 5) *(A)* versus controls (n = 5 + 5) *(B)*. > indicates higher and < lower values in the first group ($p \leqslant 0.05$). I and II denote first and second comparison, respectively.

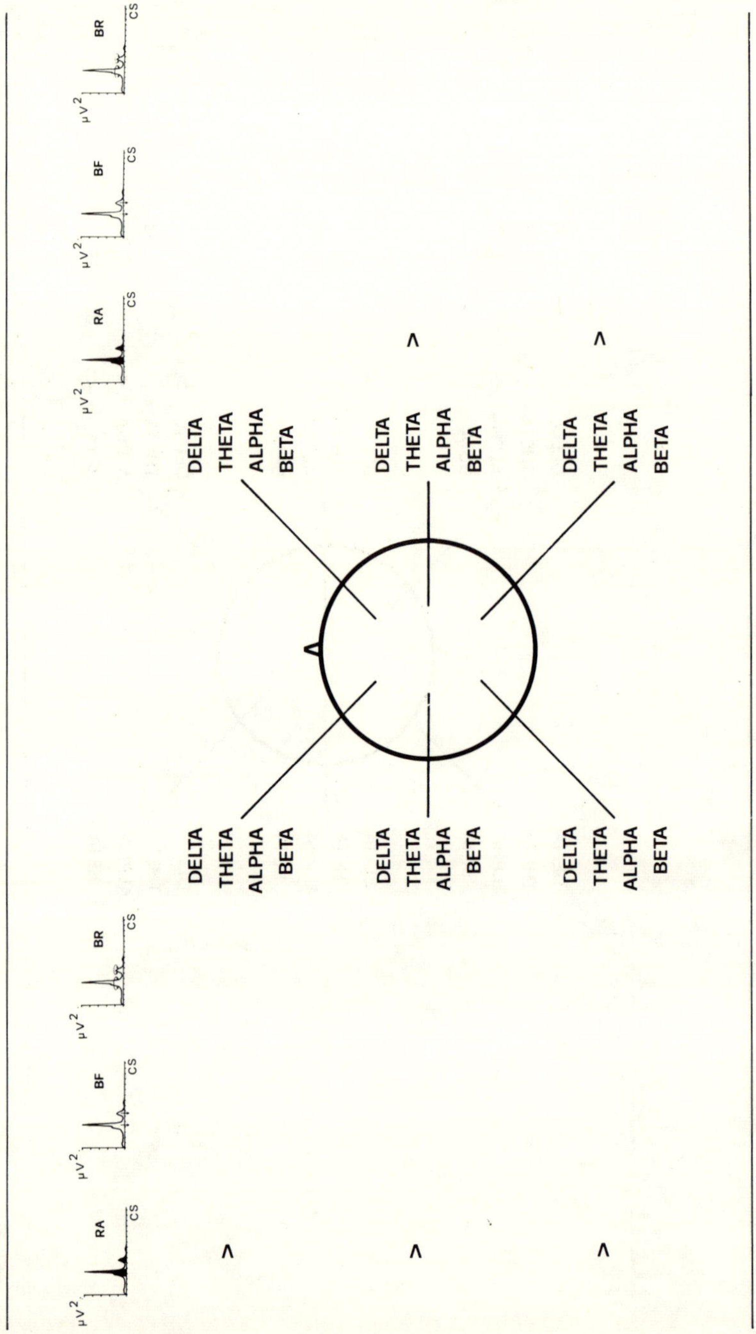

Fig. 4. Heroin addicts (n = 31) *(A)* versus controls (n = 31) *(B)*. > indicates higher and < lower values in the first group ($p \leqslant 0.05$).

Table I. EEG comparisons in schizophrenic subgroups

Group	N	EEG spectral differences
Schizophrenics vs. controls	67 65	schizophrenics alpha RA lower and beta RA, BF, BR higher in frontal, parietal leads
Chronic schizophrenics vs. Schizophrenic acute exacerbations	38 29	chronics schizophrenics theta BF higher in both frontal and parietal leads
Paranoid schizophrenics vs. controls	46 65	differences very similar to those found in the comparison between schizophrenics (67) and controls (65)
Hallucinating schizophrenics vs. controls	21 65	differences very similar to those found in the comparisons between schizophrenics (67) paranoids (46 and controls (65)
Hallucinating schizophrenics vs. nonhallucinatory schizophrenics	21 46	no significant difference
Severe autistic schizophrenics vs. no evident autism schizophrenics	20 26	no significant difference
Severe autistic schizophrenics vs. controls	20 65	autistic schizophrenics beta BF higher in both frontal and parietal leads (data found) comparing schizophrenics (67) and controls (65)

Only significant differences are indicated. The symptoms were scored according to CPRS of *Åsberg* et al. [1976]. Other schizophrenic subgroups not evaluated because of their small number. ($p \leqslant 0.05$).

sodes of acute exacerbation. Paranoid, severe autistic and hallucinatory schizophrenics, when compared with healthy controls, had EEG spectral differences very similar to those found between the whole group of schizophrenics and controls, but no significant difference occurred when the above-mentioned subgroups of schizophrenics were compared with each other (table I). Many EEG differences were noted between healthy males and females; however, very few differences were found between schizophrenic males and females (table II). Furthermore, the schizophrenic males had a large number of differences compared to healthy males, but very few differences were found between the schizophrenic females and healthy females (table II). In table II it can also be seen that the schizophrenic males showed spectral deviations mostly in the delta, theta

Table II. EEG comparisons between sexes in selected subgroups

Group	Sex	n	EEG mean spectral differences	Total
Schizophrenics vs. schizophrenics	M F	32 35	male delta RA, lower right OCC, alpha RA, higher right OCC, BF lower left OCC, BR lower right OCC, beta RA lower both PA and OCC	8
Controls vs. controls	M F	33 32	male delta RA, lower right FR, OCC, theta RA lower FR, PA, OCC, alpha RA higher FR, PA and OCC, alpha BR higher FR, PA and left OCC	19
Schizophrenics vs. controls	M M	32 33	schizophrenics delta RA higher both FR, PA and left OCC, theta RA higher both FR and PA, alpha RA lower both FR and PA, beta BF higher left FR, alpha BR higher left PA, beta BR higher both FR, PA and OCC	21
Schizophrenics vs. controls	F F	35 32	schizophrenics theta RA lower right FR, beta RA higher both FR, and PA, beta BF both FR	7
Schizophrenics vs. controls	M+F M+F	67 65	schizophrenics delta RA higher right FR, PA, left PA, alpha RA lower both FR, PA and left OCC, alpha BR lower left PA, beta BF higher both FR and PA, beta BR higher both FR, PA and OCC	19

FR = Frontal; PA = parietal; OCC = occipital. Only significant differences are indicated.

Table III. EEG interhemispheric comparisons

Controls (n = 65)		Schizophrenics (n = 67)		Depressives (n = 22)		Heroin addicts (n = 31)	
RA							
Theta frontal	R > L			delta parietal	R > L	delta parietal	R < L
Theta parietal	R > L			theta parietal	R > L	alpha parietal	R < L
				alpha parietal	R < L		
BF							
Theta occipital	R > L	alpha frontal	R < L	beta occipital	R < L		
Beta occipital	R < L	alpha parietal	R < L				
BR							
Beta occipital	R < L	alpha frontal	R < L	delta occipital	R < L		
		alpha parietal	R < L	beta frontal	R < L		
		beta occipital	R < L	beta parietal	R < L		
				beta occipital	R < L		

R = Right; L = left. Only significant differences are indicated ($p \leqslant 0.05$)

and alpha RA and the schizophrenic females in the beta RA. The differences in the beta BF and BR were more equally distributed among the males and females (table II). The healthy controls had few interhemispheric asymmetries in the theta and beta RA, BF and BR, the schizophrenics showed no asymmetries in the RA and very few interhemispheric differences condensed in the frontal and parietal alpha BF and BR that were lower in the nondominant hemisphere (table III). In general, the depressed patients had a larger number of differences between the two hemispheres. They were more condensed in slow bands RA that were higher in the right hemisphere (nondominat) and in the beta BR that was smaller in the nondominant frontal, parietal and occipital areas (table III). The heroin addicts showed the smallest number of asymmetries that were in the parietal delta and alpha RA only (table III). The serum prolactin levels were within the normal range of values in all of the subjects and no significant difference was found between the experimental groups or between males and females.

Comments

In general, the findings indicate that schizophrenics, depressives and heroin addicts have high significant EEG quantitative differences compared to healthy subjects, and suggest that brain functional deviations may be found in these psychiatric patients as well as in the chronic heroin users. In the schizophrenics, the results suggest that in these psychotics there is mostly in the frontal and parietal areas a shifting of the EEG signals from the frequencies, laying in the alpha band, to the slow bands (delta and theta) as well as to the fast frequencies (beta). These data confirm those of *Giannitrapani and Kayton* [1974], *Itil* et al. [1974], *Shagass* et al. [1979] as well as our previous findings [*Kemali* et al., 1980a, b; *Vacca* et al., 1980]. They also support the hypothesis of an increased state of cortical activation in schizophrenics [*Goldstein* et al., 1963; *Brune* 1971]. The depressed patients showed a small and dispersed number of deviations compared to controls. These findings are not fully in line with those of other investigators [*Perris* et al., 1978; *Monakhov* et al., 1979] but in this connection it has to be mentioned that the majority of subjects of our sample are neurotic-reactive depressives and that different methods have been used. The small sample of obsessional-compulsive patients showed very different EEG spectral deviations in the two consecutive comparisons with healthy controls. This result underlines the problems of the high variability of the brain bioelectric activity [*Shagass* et al., 1979] and of the EEG as a stochastic process. In our findings the spectral characteristics of heroin addicts, when compared with matched controls, indicate a cerebral functional disorganization in the left frontal and in both parietal and occipital areas. They indicate, in line with reports by other authors [*Alberti*, 1976; *Judd* et al., 1978], that it is very likely that the EEG deviations, condensed in the slow frequencies, are correlatable to the chronic abuse of opiate derivatives and that it may indicate a brain structural impairment [*Grant and Judd*, 1976; *Del Vecchio* et al., 1980], but we do not have the baseline EEG records of the heroin addicts. Furthermore, other investigators [*Lewis* et al., 1970] indicate an increased shifting to a lower stage of vigilance in the opiate users.

In our findings, symptoms as hallucinations and autism seem not to be correlatable to the EEG deviations found in the schizophrenics. The paranoid schizophrenics showed EEG deviations from normals very similar to those of the whole group of schizophrenics. Concerning this last similarity, it has to be mentioned that paranoids are the largest diagnostic subgroup (46 subjects of a total of 67 schizophrenics) and that it may be the determinant in the statistical evaluations. Comparing the chronic schizophrenics with the schizophrenic in an acute state of exacerbation the data indicate that some neurophysiological differences may exist in these two different psychopathological conditions. With respect to the variable sex, our EEG data indicate that schizophrenic males and females are subgroups more homogeneous than the healthy subjects, who in fact show many spectral differences between the two sexes. Moreover, the results also suggest that some specific spectral EEG differences between schizophrenics and controls may be linked to the sex (i.e. the beta activity more linked to the females and the alpha activity to the males). These last results are in line with those of other investigators [*Shagass* et al., 1979] and with our previous studies [*Kemali* et al., 1980a, b]. The results on the interhemispheric comparisons indicate that schizophrenics and heroin addicts have hypersymmetric EEG records. For schizophrenics the data are complementary to the 'monotonous EEG' reported by *Snezhnewsky* [1961] and 'hyperstable EEG' of *Shagass* et al. [1979]. In conclusion, our findings indicate that schizophrenics, depressives and obsessives are psychiatric patients with brain functional deviations from normals, and that chronic heroin abusers have EEG slow wave differences when compared to controls. In heroin abusers it still has to be determined if the EEG pattern may indicate a brain functional disorganization or a brain structural impairment.

Summary

Multichannel EEG records of 76 healthy volunteers, 67 schizophrenics, 22 depressives, 31 heroin addicts and 5 obsessives were collected. All of the patients had been drug-free for at least 14 days prior to EEG. Averaged power and frequency spectral parameters were calculated using relative and geometrical descriptors. Each experimental group was compared with controls comparable for number, sex and age. The results indicate that the psychiatric patients of the above-mentioned diagnostic categories and the chronic heroin users had neurophysiological brain disorganization. No significant differences were found in the serum prolactin levels.

References

Abrams, R.; Taylor, M.A.: Differential EEG patterns in affective disorder and schizophrenia. Archs gen. Psychiat. *36:* 1355–1359 (1979).

Alberti, G.: in De Maio, Le tossicomanie giovanili, pp. 203–216 (Pensiero Scientifico, Roma 1976).

Åsberg, M.; Montgomery, S.; Perris, C.; Schelling, D.; Sedvall, G.: The comprehensive psychopathological rating scale (CPRS). Annu. Meet. Scand. Soc. Psychopharm., Copenhagen 1976.

Astrachan, B.M., et al.: in Strahilevitz, Narasimbachari, Fischer, Melzer, Himwich, Indoleethilamine-N-methyltransferase activity in psychiatric patients and controls. Biol. Psychiat. *10:* 287–302 (1975).

Brune, G.G.: Somatically determined psychoses; in Himwich, Biochemistry of schizophrenia and affective illness (Williams & Wilkins, Baltimore 1971).

Del Vecchio, M.; Vacca, L.; Marciano, F.; Nolfe, G.; Iorio, G.; Maj, M.; Kemali, D.: Biochemical and CEEG investigation in drug addicts: preliminary findings; in Richter, Addiction and brain damage, pp. 240–255 (Croom Helm, London 1980).

Feighner, J.P.; Robins, E.; Guze, S.B.; Woodruff, R.; Winokur, K.; Munor, R.: Diagnostic criteria for use in psychiatric research. Archs gen. Psychiat. *26:* 57–63 (1972).

Flor-Henry, P.; Koles, Z.J.; Howarth, B.G.; Burton, L.: Neurophysiological studies of schizophrenia, mania and depression; in Grouzelier, Flor-Henry, Hemisphere asymmetries of function in psychopathology, pp. 189–222 (Elsevier/North-Holland, Amsterdam 1979a).

Flor-Henry, P.; Yendall, L.T.; Koles, Z.J.; Howarth, B.G.: Neuropsychological and power spectral EEG investigation of the obsessive-compulsive syndrome. Biol. Psychiat. *14:* 119–129 (1979b).

Franzen, G.; Ingvar, D.H.: Abnormal distribution of cerebral activity in chronic schizophrenia. J. psychiat. Res. *12:* 199–214 (1975).

Giannitrapani, O.; Kayton, L.: Schizophrenia and EEG spectrum analysis. Electroenceph. clin. Neurophysiol. *36:* 377–386 (1974).

Goldstein, L.; Murphree, H.B.; Sugerman, A.; Pfeiffer, C.: Quantitative elektroencephalographic analysis of naturally and drug-induced psychotic states in human males. Clin. Pharmacol. Ther. *4:* 10–21 (1963).

Grant, I.; Judd, L.: Neurophysiological and EEG disturbances in polydrug users. Am. J. Psychiat. *133:* 1039–1042 (1976).

Gur, R.E.: Cognitive concomitants of hemispheric dysfunction in schizophrenia. Archs gen. Psychiat. *36:* 269–274 (1979).

Hwang, P.; Guyda, H.; Friesen, H.: A radioimmunoassay for human prolactin. Proc. nath. Acad. Sci USA *68:* 1902–1906 (1971).

Itil, T.; Saletu, B.; Davis, S.: Stability studies in schizophrenics and normals using computer-analyzed EEG. Biol. Psychiat. *8:* 321–335 (1974).

Judd, L.; Grant, I.; Bickford, R.G.; Lee, W.G.: in Wesson, Carlin, Adams, Beschner, Polydrug abuse: the results of a national collaborative study, pp. 273–297 (Academic Press, New York 1978).

Kemali, D.; Vacca, L.; Marciano, F.; Celani, T.; Nolfe, G.; Iorio, G.: Computerized EEG in schizophrenics. Neuropsychobiology *6:* 260–267 (1980a).

Kemali, D.; Vacca, L.; Nolfe, G.; Iorio, G.; De Carlo, R.: Hemispheric EEG quantitative asymmetries in schizophrenics and depressed patients. Adv. biol. Psychiat., vol. 4, pp. 14–20 (Karger, Basel 1980b).

Lewis, E.G.; Oswald, I.; Evans, S.I.; Akindala, M.; Tompset, S.L.: Heroin and human sleep. Electroenceph. clin. Neurophysiol. *28:* 374–381 (1970).

Marciano, F.; Nolfe, G.: Pattern recognition of biomedical aspects (Quaderni della ricerca scientifica del CNR-108, 1980).

Monakhov, K.; Perris, C.; Botskarev, K.; Knorring, L. von; Nikiforov, A.I.: Functional interhemispheric differences in relation to various psychopathological components of depressive syndromes. Neuropsychobiology *5:* 143–155 (1979).

Perris, C.: A study of bipolar and unipolar depressive psychoses. Acta psychiat. scand. *42:* suppl. 194, pp. 118–152 (1966).

Perris, C.; Monakhov, K.; Knorring, L. von; Botskarev, K.: System structural analysis of electroencephalogram in depressed patients. General principles and preliminary results of an international collaborative study. Neuropsychobiology *4:* 193–266 (1978).

Raczkowsky, O.; Kalat, J.W.; Mebes, R.: Reliability and validity of some handedness questionnaire items. Neuropsychologia *12:* 43–47 (1974).

Schneider, K.: Psicopatologia generale, pp. 94–96 (Sansoni, Firenze 1966).

Shagass, C.; Straumanis, D.; Overton, D.A.: Correlations between psychiatric diagnoses and some quantitative EEG variables. Neuropsychobiology *5:* 16–26 (1979).

Snezhnewsky, A.V.: Psychopharmacology, the pathophysiology of higher nervous activity and clinical psychiatry. Ann. N.Y. Acad. Sci. *92:* 813–1198 (1961).

Vacca, L.; Kemali, D.; Marciano, F.; Celani, T.; Pierro, C.: Quantitative EEG analysis in schizophrenia and depressed patients. Adv. Biol. Psychiat. *4:* 111–118 (1980).

D. Kemali, MD, Clinica Psichiatrica, Prima Facoltà di Medicina e Chirurgia, Università di Napoli, Piazza Miraglia, 2, I-80138 Napoli (Italia)

Adv. biol. Psychiat., vol. 6, pp. 29–34 (Karger, Basel 1981)

Schizophrenia Assessed by Computerized EEG[1]

P. Etevenon, P. Peron-Magnan, P. Rioux, B. Pidoux, J.C. Bisserbe, G. Verdeaux, P. Deniker[2]

Section d'EEG Quantitative du Service Hospitalo-Universitaire de Santé Mentale et de Thérapeutique et Service d'Exploration Fonctionnelle du Système Nerveux, Centre Hospitalier Sainte-Anne, Paris, France

Stat crux dum volvitur orbis.
Ernst Jünger, Heliopolis, 1949

In the scientific literature, quantitative computerized electroencephalography methods, applied to EEGs of schizophrenic patients, have provided four main findings: (1) Hypovariability, hyperstability of EEGs [1, 3, 4, 9–11, 13–16] expressed by low coefficients of variation (CV) of total mean amplitude (a_t) and/or mean frequency (f_t). (2) Specific features of EEGs of 'paranoid type' patients [3, 8, 10, 11, 13, 14]: lower a_t and f_t, higher amplitudes for low and fast frequency rhythms. (3) Specific features of EEGs of 'residual type' patients (hebephrenic patients) [2–4, 8, 10, 11, 13, 14]: higher a_t and f_t, highly stable alpha peak. (4) EEG amplitude changes: hemispheric asymmetries between absolute values of amplitudes of raw EEG [1, 3, 4, 6, 7]. The left/right occipital amplitude ratio is greater than 1.5 for EEGs of schizophrenic patients. However, this is not the case when considering the relative values of amplitudes (expressed in terms of percentage power density); the left/right ratio becoming nearby unity [12, 16, 17].

These findings have been verified on small groups of schizophrenic patients (n = 43, average number from 15 articles, range 10–101) divided into subgroups even smaller (an average of 10 hebephrenic patients, 17 paranoid patients and 11 'others' when considering 7 published articles). Then, the problem remains of differentiating between subgroups of schizophrenic patients and checking the stability of previous findings [2, 3] when increasing the number of patients. Another problem will be also to compare EEGs of schizophrenic patients with EEGs of normal volunteers and/or EEGs of others psychotic patients.

[1] This work was supported by INSERM Research Grants ATP 65.78.97 and ATP 73.79.105 and UER Cochin-Port-Royal.

[2] We wish to thank Mr. *Letel* for his skilful EEG recordings and Fourier analysis management. We are grateful to Miss *Guillou* for endless statistical data treatment.

Table I. Sample: schizophrenic patients, n = 34

Type of patients	R: Residual	O: Others	P: Paranoid
Number of patients	n = 11 (1F)	n = 16 (1F)	n = 7
Age (19–44), years,	25.5	26.5	28.4
CV, %	29.7	20.6	16.1
Duration of illness (0.7–15), years	5	4.3	6
r	0.88**	0.44$^{(*)}$	0.84**
F	29.8**	3.4$^{(*)}$	11.9*

$p \leqslant 0.01$**; $p \leqslant 0.05$*; $p \leqslant 0.10^{(*)}$

Patients and Methods

The criteria of *Feighner* et al. [5] have been applied to our clinical material for selecting 34 recorded patients as schizophrenics. Moreover, complementary criteria have been used, based on DSM-3, differentiating 3 subgroups: 'residual type' (R), 'paranoid type' (P), and 'others' (O) which can be either (R + P) mixed type of schizophrenia or classified under other headings of the DSM-3. 7 of the patients were treated with neuroleptics (4 'P', 3 'O') at the time of EEG recording, the remaining patients were free for 1 week of treatment.

In table I are indicated the number of patients in each of the three subgroups, the mean ages with CVs, the mean duration of illness. The coefficient of correlation r between age and duration of illness is greater for R and P than for O subgroup. The test F of linearity has also been expressed in table I. This indicates a greater dispersion in age and duration of illness for subgroup O compared to R and P. In comparison with this group of patients, we have recorded 47 EEGs in 31 normal volunteers. This group of control was matched in age with the group of patients.

The recording protocol has been already published [3, 4]. 5 min of EEG were recorded in a relaxed situation, the subject or patient being seated, the eyes closed. Four EEG channels were recorded simultaneously: C4-P4, P4-O2, C3-P3, and P3-O1, sampled at 200 Hz every 2.56 s. The methods of statistical spectral analysis of EEG have also been published in detail [3, 4]. After a double rejection of artifacts, the sampled EEGs are stored on disc. The Fourier Analyser (hp 5451 B equiped with 2100 S microprogrammable computer, disc, digital tape recorder, and peripheral outputs) is performing on-line digitalization of EEG, followed by computations of evolutive power spectra, average power spectra and spectral variances, cross-spectra, and coherences between the four EEG channels. Spectral t-tests provide statistical comparisons between 2 autospectra. This is followed by data reduction depicted in table II.

Statistical multivariate analysis is computed off-line at the CITI 2 computer center. A first quadratic discriminant analysis, step by step method is applied to the data base made of 84 characteristic spectral parameters computed for each EEG recording of schizophrenic sample EEGs and/or normal control volunteer EEGs. A second principal component analysis followed by cluster analysis is then computed on the same data base. This last arborescent hierarchical classification method is using a locally adaptive clustering algorithm.

Table II. Data reduction: characteristic spectral parameters from 24 to 248 parameters; 5 min of EEG, 4 channels

Mean frequency (centroid): δ, Θ, α, β 1, β 2, total
Coefficient of variation (CV)
Mobility (Hjorth)

Mean amplitude (μV): δ, Θ, α, β 1, β 2, total
Coefficient of variation (CV)
Amplitude ratios (dissymmetry)

Mean relative amplitude (%): δ, Θ, α, β 1, β 2,
Standard deviation

Resonance coefficient k (1 sine wave, 0.1 noise)
Theta/alpha ratio

Parameters used for multivariate analysis (≤ 84)

Table III. Results

1 *Hypovariability* (discriminant analysis)
CV amplitude C3–P3
25.3% (P) < 28.7% (R) < 34.3% (O)
28.9% (P+R+O) < 35.8% (normals)

2 *Paranoid type* (Mann-Whitney test)
Lower alpha amplitude
Lower mean frequency * $p \leq 0.05$
Higher theta %
Better discriminated than residual type and/or others EEG groups

3 *Classification*
First two clusters
High alpha %
Low alpha %
in (P+R+O) and/or in normals

Results

Table III presents the three main findings of this study. First, the hypovariability of EEGs of schizophrenic patients is well quantified by the coefficient of variation of left centro-parietal amplitudes. This is the first discriminant coefficient (table IV, V). Secondly, the paranoid type of EEGs presents specific features when compared to R and O subgroups of EEGs. Finally, the classification method distinguishes two first clusters: high and low alpha percentage EEGs. These two clusters are found in the group of pathological EEGs as well as in the group of normal EEGs.

Table IV. Quadratic discriminant analysis (34 EEGs of schizophrenic patients)

Variable	Definition
1	CV (amplitude alpha C3–P3)
2	Mean frequency (theta P3–01)
3	Mean amplitude (beta 1, C4–P4)
4	Mean amplitude (beta 1, C3–P3)
5	CV (amplitude delta P4–02)
6	Mean frequency (beta 1, C4–P4)

Table V. Quadratic discriminant analysis (34 EEGs of schizophrenic patients)

Variables /groups	Sensitivity, %			Predicitive value, %		
	R	O	P	R	O	P
1	82	50	71	60	88	50
2	73	75	86	72	92	60
3	73	88	*100*	80	82	*100*
4	82	*100*	*100*	*100*	88	*100*
5	91	*100*	*100*	*100*	94	*100*
6	*100*	*100*	*100*	*100*	*100*	*100*

Residual type R is the least well recognized group;
others O is the least well predicted group;
paranoid type P is the best discriminated group.

Table IV presents the results of the quadratic discriminant analysis which provides a total discrimination between the three subgroups of pathological EEGs after taking into account six parameters. Table V presents the computed values of sensitivity percentage and predictive value percentage after introducing step by step a new variable. We have observed that the paranoid type group of EEGs is the best discriminated group when compared to the other two subgroups R and O.

Discussion

In these results we have verified again the hypovariability of EEGs of schizophrenic patients, the specific features of the paranoid subgroup especially, but not the hemispheric amplitude changes. This last negative finding may be explained by a different sample of EEGs. Our previous study [3] was done with a small number of patients who were very homogeneous, and where multiple EEG recordings were taken into account, instead of one EEG recording for every patient in this present study.

The discriminant analysis result is better in this study than in the preceding one [3]; 84 variables (table II) are used instead of 24 variables. Nevertheless, the classification based on cluster analysis is less demonstrative in that study than in the first one [2]; a greater number of variables may have produced some 'noise' blurring the results of this classification.

Despite the specific technical problems of multivariate analysis, the nonparametric Mann-Whitney statistic used for comparing characteristic spectral parameters between couples of the three subgroups (P-O, P-R, R-O) reveals significant statistical changes between R-P and also O-P, but not between O and R subgroups. Then the EEGs of the P subgroup are lower in absolute amplitude (RMS value), lower in mean frequency, and present a greater theta rhythm percentage amplitude than O and R EEGs. These results are consistent with previous findings [4, 9, 11, 13–15].

Finally remains the problem of comparing EEGs of schizophrenics with other EEGs. The first two clusters provided by the classification analysis were quite similar between (R + O + P) group and the N group of control EEGs. This confirms our first classification analysis [2] where the 'high-alpha' cluster from the control group was closer to the hebephrenic subgroup cluster. Similarly with our present finding, the 'low-alpha' cluster from the control group in our first study [2] was also closer to the paranoid subgroup cluster. However, in this study the overlapping between the normal volunteers' EEG clusters and the clusters obtained from the EEGs of schizophrenic patients was greater than in our first classification [2], based on a smaller sample of patients and subjects. That remains an open problem of defining proper control groups [8] and proper amounts of patients versus subjects.

Summary

A first sample of 34 EEGs of schizophrenic patients was studied. They were classified as 'paranoid type' P (n = 7), 'residual type' R (n = 11), 'others' O (n = 16) according to Feighner's and DSM-3 criteria. A second sample of 47 EEGs recorded from 31 normal volunteers was chosen as a control group N. Statistical Fourier spectral analysis was performed in 5 min of EEG recorded under the eyes-closed condition, over 4 channels: C4-P4, P4-O2, C3-P3, P3-O1.

Hypovariability of EEGs of the first sample was confirmed by quadratic discriminant analysis: 25% of coefficient of variation for C3-P3 amplitude of the P group against 36% for the N group. The P group presented specific features compared to R and O groups: lower-alpha amplitude and mean frequency, higher theta percentage, better discriminated group. Cluster analysis revealed in the first sample and second samples: a high alpha percentage cluster and a low alpha percentage cluster, the last one overlapping the P group in the first sample.

References

1 d'Elia, G.; Jacobsson, L.; Knorring, L. von; Matisson, B.; Mjörndal, T.; Oreland, I.; Perris, C.; Rapp, W.: Changes in psychopathology in relation to EEG variables and visual averaged evoked responses (V. AER) in schizophrenic patients treated with penfluridol or thiothixene. Acta psychiat. scand. *55:* 309–318 (1977).

2 Etevenon, P.; Pidoux, B.; Rioux, P.: Strategy of statistical spectral analysis in drug studies. A methological synopsis; in Saletu, Neuropsychopharmacology, pp. 383–391 (Pergamon Press, Oxford 1979).

3 Etevenon, P.; Pidoux, B.; Rioux, P.; Peron-Magnan, P.; Verdeaux, G.; Deniker, P.: Intra- and interhemispheric EEG differences quantified by spectral analysis. Acta psychiat. scand. *60:* 57–68 (1979).

4 Etevenon, P.; Pidoux, B.; Cottereau, M.J.; Peron-Magnan, P.; Zarifian, E.; Verdeaux, G.; Deniker, P.: Quantitative EEG analysis of high-dosage haloperidol effects in therapy-resistant schizophrenic patients. Adv. biol. Psychiat. vol. 4, pp. 175–187 (Karger, Basel 1980).

5 Feighner, J.P.; Robins, E.; Guze, S.B.; Woodruff, R.A.; Winokur, G.; Munoz, R.: Diagnostic criteria for use in psychiatric research. Archs gen. Psychiat. *26:* 57–63 (1972).

6 Flor-Henry, P.: Lateralized temporal-limbic dysfunction and psychopathology. Ann. N.Y. Acad. Sci. *280:* 777–795 (1976).

7 Flor-Henry, P.; Koles, Z.J.: EEG studies in depression, mania and normals: evidence for partial shifts of laterality in the affective psychoses. Adv. biol. Psychiat., vol. 4, pp. 21–43 (Karger, Basel 1980).

8 Fink, M.; Itil, T.M.; Clyde, D.: The classification of psychoses by quantitative EEG measures; in Wortis, Recent advances in biological psychiatry, vol. 8, pp. 305–312 (Plenum Press, New York 1966).

9 Goldstein, L.; Sugerman, A.A.; Stolberg, H.; Murphree, H.B.; Pfeiffer, C.C.: Electrocerebral activity in Schizophrenics and non psychotic subjects, quantitative EEG amplitude analysis. Electroenceph. clin. Neurophysiol. *19:* 350–361 (1965).

10 Itil, T.M.: Qualitative and quantitative EEG findings in schizophrenia. Schiz. Bull. *3:* 61–78 (1977).

11 Itil, T.M.; Saletu, B.; Davis, S.: EEG findings in chronic scizophrenics based on digital computer period analysis and analog power spectra. Biol. Psychiat. *5:* 1 (1972).

12 Kemali, D.; Vacca, L.; Nolfe, G.; Iorio, G.; De Carlo, R.: Hemispheric EEG quantitative asymmetries in schizophrenics and depressed patients. Adv. biol. Psychiat., vol. 4, pp. 14–20 (Karger, Basel 1980).

13 Lifshitz, K.; Gradijan, J. Relationships between measures of the coefficient of variation of the mean absolute EEG voltage and spectral intensities in schizophrenic and control subjects. Biol. Psychiat. *5:* 149–163 (1972).

14 Lifshitz, K.; Gradijan, J.: Spectral evaluation of the electroencephalogram: power and variability in chronic schizophrenics and control subjects. Psychophysiology *11:* 479–490 (1974).

15 Marjerrisson, G.; Krause, A.E.; Keogh, R.P.: Variability of the EEG in schizophrenia. Quantitative analysis with a modulus voltage integrator. Electroenceph. clin. Neurophysiol. *24:* 35–41 (1968).

16 Pidoux, B.; Peron-Magnan, P.; Etevenon, P.; Verdeaux, G.; Deniker, P.: L'activité alpha dans un groupe de schizophrènes: analyse spectrale et comparaison avec un groupe témoin. Rev. Electroencéphalogr. Neurophysiol. clin. *8:* 283–293 (1978).

17 Vacca, L.; Kemali, D.; Marciano, F.; Celani, T.; Pierro, C.: Quantitative EEG analysis in schizophrenics and depressed patients. Adv. biol. Psychiat., vol. 4, pp. 111–118 (Karger, Basel 1980).

P. Etevenon, DSc, Inserm, 2 Rue d'Alésia, F–75014 Paris (France)

Adv. biol. Psychiat., vol. 6, pp. 35–40 (Karger, Basel 1981)

EEG and Behavioral Differences between First Acute Schizophrenic Episode and Remission

Martha Koukkou[1]

Research Department, Psychiatric University Hospital, Zürich, Switzerland

Introduction

Our research in schizophrenia is centered around studies of the EEG characteristics of the orienting response in acute and former schizophrenics. It has been assumed that if the orienting reaction is a fundamental mechanism of the organism for its communication with the environment [1], the schizophrenic communication and performance deficit [2] may be reflected in a deviation of the EEG correlates of the orienting reaction.

In an information processing approach the appearence or omission of an orienting reaction as a consequence of incoming information is the execution of a selected response after a series of perceptual and cognitive operations: sensory excitation, short-term storage, comparison of input with long-term storages, response selection and execution [3]. Studies of the EEG correlates of information processing indicate that the characteristics of EEG reactivity to inputs (EEG characteristics of the orienting response) reflect the 'initial interpretation' of the information by the central nervous system. This reactivity introduces the brain state during which the subsequent 'full interpretation' will occur [4].

The hypothesis for these studies has been that if the productive symptoms of acute schizophrenics are due to a deviation in one or more stages of information processing, then acute schizophrenics should have an EEG reactivity to stimuli which differs from the EEG reactivity of normal controls, and of former schizophrenics during complete remission.

On the other hand, if acute and former schizophrenics show similar EEG reactivity to stimuli, and if this reactivity differed from that of normal controls, then the deviant EEG reactivity of acute and former schizophrenics would indi-

[1] I want to thank Mr. *W. Manske* and *B. Bultmann* for technical and statistical assistance and Miss *R. Rüttimann* for assistance in the preparation of the manuscript.

cate a predisposition to such symptoms but not a physiological concomitant of the symptoms.

The first steps of analysis in these studies on schizophrenic EEG reactivity to stimuli indicate that indeed acute drug-free schizophrenics have a different (ectropic) EEG reactivity to information input as compared with normals and former schizophrenics [5].

In this article I present some further characteristics of the ectropic EEG reactivity of acute schizophrenics, the results of the continuous performance test and of the time estimation test on our populations, and interpretations of the results.

Material, Method and Results

The subjects were 22 acute schizophrenics, 20 former schizophrenics, and 20 normal controls. All subjects were drug-free; the acute schizophrenics were recorded during their first schizophrenic episode, and before any psychopharmacological treatment was initiated. The criteria of the selection of a patient in the group of ***acute schizophrenics***, of ***former schizophrenics*** and of ***normal controls*** as well as the EEG recording procedure are described elsewhere [5].

The EEG part of the study was designed to yield several EEG epochs after the presentation of auditory information (conditions) to which the subjects were asked to attend. These informations consisted of: (a) the instruction to open and after 20 s to close the eyes, (b) of four randomly presented meaningless sentences made up from regular words, and (c) of 10 randomly presented short tones to which the subjects had to react with a key press. All recordings were with eyes closed except during the instruction to open the eyes.

The EEG was analyzed into power spectra, using a Fourier transformation with a program written by *H.H. Stassen;* the data were analyzed in segments of 20 s.

For reduction of the resulting frequency distributions into few descriptors, distribution means ['centroids'; 6] for the conventional clinical EEG frequency bands as well as for frequency bands based on results of principal component analysis [7] were computed. The centroid values reflect the shape of the power spectra, and are independent of total power within the analyzed band. For each subject, each condition and each frequency band the EEG reactivity was computed, defined as the amount of change of the centroids between the 80 s of resting EEG (baseline) and 20 s of EEG after each presentation. These changes were computed in intrasubject comparisons and were expressed as one value per subject, condition and frequency band. Since the computation uses each subject as its own control, these difference values establish common EEG characteristics of the induced change for all subjects within each group, regardless of the idiosyncratic characteristics of the individual resting EEG activity. This procedure implies the avoidance of the usual EEG problem of excessive variance of baseline values between subjects.

In this paper we consider the EEG reactivity between baseline and the eye-closing conditions, and the two first sentences measured with the 2–8 and 9–13 Hz centroids of the left parieto-occipital lead. All subjects were self-reported right handers.

After the EEG recordings the subjects were asked to estimate the time duration of the EEG recording and then to participate in a continuous performance test (CPT, auditory stimuli). For the group of acute schizophrenics these results will be omitted from further analysis because of the large number of errors of omission.

Table I. Mean, standard deviation and p values of number of missing and wrong responses on the CPT; reaction time to the 80·stimuli of PTC and to 10 tones and time estimation

	Former schizophrenics		Controls		
Performance	X	SD	X	SD	p
CPT omissions	1.45	2.03	1.75	3.27	n.s.
CPT errors	3.80	5.67	2.80	4.80	n.s.
CPT reaction time, ms	472	149	392	69	0.02
Tones reaction time, ms	367	119	428	75	n.s.
Time estimation, %	59.05	26	80.75	25	0.02

Table II. p values of comparisons of EEG reactivity between the three groups; the three stimuli and the two EEG centroids. C = controls; A = acute schizophrenics; F = former schizophrenics

	p values t-test								
	eyes			sentence 1			sentence 2		
Centroid	C/A	C/F	F/A	C/A	C/F	F/A	C/A	C/F	F/A
2–8	0.00	0.01	n.s.	n.s.	n.s.	n.s.	n.s.	n.s.	n.s.
9–13	0.00	n.s.	0.01	0.08	n.s.	0.00	0.04	n.s.	0.00

Univariate analysis of variance was carried out on each of the EEG variables and each of the EEG reactivity measures. The significance of the difference in EEG reactivity and behavior between groups was tested with t-test and unpaired Man-Whitney U-test, respectively.

Table I shows the results of the behavioral data for the former schizophrenics and the controls, indicating that there is no significant difference between these two groups in the number of omissions or errors on the CPT. The two groups are however distinctly different in reaction time to CPT stimuli and in time estimation. The former schizophrenics show longer mean reaction times and estimate a time unit shorter than normals. The mean reaction time of the former schizophrenics to the initially presented ten tones is not significantly different from the reaction time of the controls although numerically shorter.

Table II and figure 1 show the EEG results. It is clear that the amount of change of the 2–8 Hz centroid from baseline to the states after the presentation of the 3 stimuli is similar for all three groups, except for the eye-closing condition, where normals react significantly stronger than the two other groups ($p = 0.00$ and $\eta^2 = 14\%$ in ANOVA, and $p < .01$ in t-test between normals and the two other groups). In the 9–13 Hz alpha band, however, there is

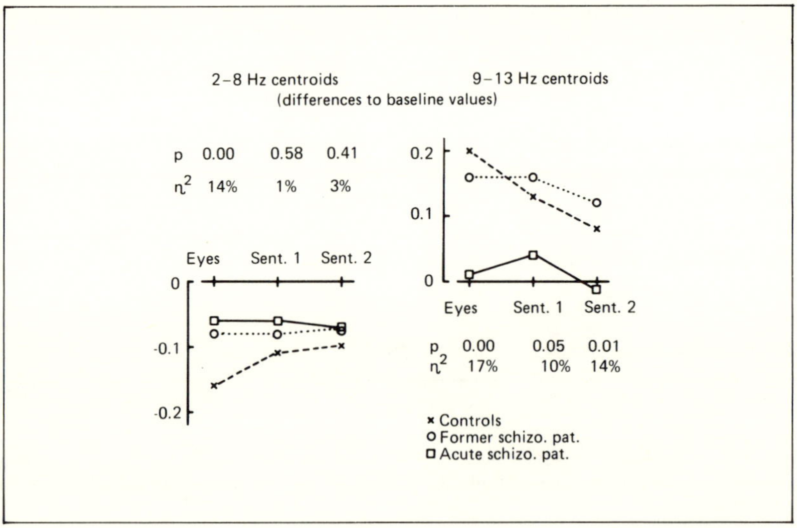

Fig. 1. Mean values of EEG changes (differences, vertical) for the 2–8 and 9–13 Hz frequency bands in the three subject groups, and the three stimuli, p and η^2 values of ANOVA are shown.

no significant difference in the EEG reactivity between normals and former schizophrenics but there are distinct differences between acute schizophrenics on the one hand and normals and former schizophrenics on the other hand. In summary, these results show that the EEG reactivity to stimuli (defined as the amount of difference between the EEG baseline and the EEG state after stimulus presentation) is similar in normal controls and former schizophrenics, but strikingly different in acute schizophrenics. Acute schizophrenics react in an ectropic way to the incoming information since they react mainly with the slow waves.

Discussion

The concept of our EEG studies on schizophrenia is based on an extended model of the brain mechanisms of information processing [4, 8] which considers different brain states with associated EEG manifestations as decisive for information processing, in particular for the late stages, i.e. for the stages of comparison of the input with long-term memory, which leads to the 'initial interpretation' of the information and the election of the initial response [3]. The state introduced by this response, in turn, is decisive for the 'full interpretation' of the information. According to the model different functional states of the brain are associated with different cognitive strategies, e.g. wakeful adult thinking, child fantasies, dream cognition [9] and with access to different memory storages [state-dependent learning and memory; 10]. Different functional states are also associated with different EEG characteristics [9]. Thus, according to this model, the ectropic EEG reactivities to the incoming informations found in our acute schizophrenics lead to the consequence that received informations are compared during full interpretation with memory contents and treated with strategies and decision tactics which are different from the ones used by former schizophrenics and normals.

These results [5] cannot help deciding whether the ectropic EEG reactivity of the acute schizophrenics is the result of a wrongly selected response or of a wrong execution of a correctly selected response. In both cases however, according to the model, received informations will have to be treated with strategies and be compared with memory storages which are not identical with the ones used by normals.

Since the EEG reactivity of former schizophrenics was found to be similar to that of normals and different to that of acute schizophrenics, the data support the hypothesis that the ectropic EEG reactivity reflects or correlates with the productive symptoms of schizophrenia and does not indicate a predisposition to the symptoms. Contrarily, the longer reaction times and the different time estimation of the group of former schizophrenics seem to confirm, in the symptom-free population, the frequent finding in schizophrenia of slower reaction times [for review, see 11] and of a deviation in time estimation [12] indicating that possibly these two findings demonstrate a characteristic of schizophrenia which is independent of the productive symptoms.

Summary

Reaction time, time estimation, and EEG recordings during resting and after stimuli were obtained in drug-free acute and former schizophrenics and normals. EEG power spectra reduced to centroids. The amount of change of the centroids between baseline and EEG after each stimulus was computed. Normals and former schizophrenics showed a similar EEG reactivity. Acute schizophrenics reacted only with the delta-theta centroid, indicating an ectropic brain state during information processing which is detectable only in the presence of productive symptoms. Contrarily time estimation and reaction time differentiated normals from former schizophrenics, indicating schizophrenic characteristics in the symptom-free patient group.

References

1 Sokolov, E.N.: Higher nervous functions: the orienting reflex. Ann. Rev. Physiol. *25:* 545–580 (1963).

2 Chapman, L.J.: Recent advances in the study of schizophrenic cognition. Schiz. Bull. *5:* 568–580 (1979).

3 Atkinson, R.C.; Shiffrin, R.M.: Human memory: a proposed system and its control processes; in Spence, Spence, The psychology of learning and motivation, vol. II (Academic Press, New York 1968).

4 Koukkou, M.; Lehmann, D.: Psychophysiologie des Träumens und der Neurosentherapie: Das Zustands-Wechsel-Modell, eine Synopsis. Fortschr. Neurol. Psychiat. *48:* 324–350 (1980).

5 Koukkou, M.: EEG reactivity in acute schizophrenics reflects deviant (ectropic) state changes during information processing; in Koukkou, Lehmann, Angst, Functional states of the brain: their determinants, pp. 265–290 (Elsevier, Amsterdam 1980).

6 Lehmann, D.; Koukkou, M.: Computer analysis of EEG wakefulness sleep patterns during learning of novel and familiar sentences. Electroenceph. clin. Neurophysiol. *37:* 73–84 (1974).

7 Dolce, G.; Waldeier, H.: Spectral and multivariate analysis of EEG changes during mental activity in man. Electroenceph. clin. Neurophysiol. *36:* 577–584 (1974).

8 Koukkou, M.; Lehmann, D.: Brain functional states: determinants, constraints and implications; in Koukkou, Lehmann, Angst, Functional states of the brain: their determinants, pp. 13–20 (Elsevier, Amsterdam 1980).

9 Lehmann, D.: Fluctuations of functional state: EEG patterns, and perceptual and cognitivestrategies; in Koukkou, Lehmann, Angst, Functional states of the brain: their determinants, pp. 189–202 (Elsevier, Amsterdam 1980).

10 Overton, D.A.: Discriminative control of behavior by drug states; in Thompson, Pickens, Stimulus properties of drugs, pp. 87–110 (Appleton Century Crofts, New York 1971).

11 Neuchterlein, K.H.: Reaction time and attention in schizophrenia: a critical evaluation of the data and theories. Schiz. Bull. *3:* 373–428 (1977).

12 King, H.E.: Anticipatory behavior: temporal matching by normal and psychotic subjects. J. Psychol. *53:* 425–440 (1962).

Martha Koukkou, MD, Research Department, Psychiatric University Hospital, Lenggstrasse 31, Postfach 68, CH-8029 Zürich 8 (Switzerland)

Adv. biol. Psychiat., vol. 6, pp. 41–49 (Karger, Basel 1981)

Further Studies of Depressed Patients by Means of Computerized EEG[1]

C. Perris, L. von Knorring, J. Cumberbatch, F. Marciano

Department of Psychiatry, University of Umeå, Umeå Data Center, University of Umeå, Umeå, Sweden; Institute of Cybernetics, Naples, Italy

EEG in Depression

In previous studies concerning possible neurophysiological correlates of depressive symptomatology, we have been able to demonstrate low mean integrated amplitude (MIA), low within patient variance (WPV), low amplitudes of evoked potentials (EP) to visual stimuli and pronounced interhemispheric differences with a tendency to reduced left/right (L/R) ratios during depression [for a review, see *Perris,* 1980]. Furthermore, in studies where systemic structural analysis of the EEG was applied, the results indicated that the relationship between mental activity and neurophysiological variables is very complex. It is further complicated by a possible differential involvement of different brain areas and the correlations found are not with clinical diagnoses or clinical syndromes but with separate symptoms and signs [*Monakhov* et al., 1979].

However, in earlier studies we did not apply any kind of spectral analysis. Since we were interested to check if our findings were generalizable to other methods of investigation and as promising results concerning depressed patients have been found by means of a computer program using geometrical spectral descriptors of the EEG [*Marciano and Nolfe,* 1977; *Kemali* et al., 1980], this program has been applied to our patient series as a part of an international collaborative study. Thus, the purpose of the present study has been to summarize our first results concerning age correlations, sex differences, differences between healthy volunteers and depressed patients as well as the interhemispheric differences found in healthy volunteers and in depressed patients.

[1] Supported in part by Grants 2568 and 5740 from the Swedish Medical Research Council. The skilful technical assistance of Ms. *Sonja Holmgren* is gratefully acknowledged.

Methodology

Patient Series. The series of depressed patients included 40 patients, 16 male and 24 female with a mean age of 46.5 years (range 23–69 years). All were right-handed as ascertained with a dominance test battery suggested by *d'Elia* [1970]. 22 patients had unipolar or bipolar affective psychosis, 13 had neurotic-reactive depression and 5 had depression NUD according to the diagnostic criteria earlier presented elsewhere [*Perris,* 1966; *d'Elia* et al., 1974]. 19 of the patients had a depressive disorder of a psychotic dimension (i.e. disturbed evaluation of reality) and 21 patients had depressive disorders of a non-psychotic dimension. The patients were rated by means of the comprehensive psychopathological rating scale (CPRS) [*Asberg* et al., 1978]. The total depression score did not differ significantly between the patients with psychotic and non-psychotic depressive disorders (36.6 ± 2.9 and 30.8 ± 2.4, respectively, t = 1.53 n.s.). 18 of the patients were completely drug-free while 22 of the patients had received small and irregular dosis of tricyclics or minor tranquilizers during the last week (corresponding to imipramine less than 50 mg a day or diazepam less than 10 mg a day occasionally).

The group of healthy volunteers had the same sex distribution and the same mean age. The series included 8 males and 12 females with a mean age of 46.2 years (range 26–64 years). They were all right-handed. They had never suffered from depressive disorders. They were physically and psychiatrically healthy and completely drug-free.

EEG Recordings. The EEG recordings were made at about the same time in the morning by the same well-trained technician. The instructions to the healthy volunteers and the depressed patients were standardized. EEG was derived from six unipolar leads placed at F3, F4, C3, C4, 01 and 02 according to the international 10–20 system with left and right ear as the reference, respectively. At least 5 min of artefact-free FEG was collected with the patient in a half-reclined resting position with the eyes closed.

EEG Processing. The EEG was stored in an analogue tape recorder. Afterwards the EEG was plotted on paper and a careful check for artefacts was made. At least 40 epochs, each of 3.8 s duration, of artefact-free recordings were analogue-digital converted and a Fourier transform was applied. For further analysis the spectra were divided into four frequency bands (delta, theta, alpha and beta). Frequencies lower than 2 cps and higher than 32 cps were rejected.

The geometrical spectral descriptors as proposed by *Marciano and Nolfe* [1977] include for each frequency band the relative activity (relative mean power), the barycentric frequency (weighted mean frequency) and the barycentric radius (mean band width). However, as our first results emerged it was found that differences in the variability of the frequency spectra could occur without being detected by means of these spectral descriptors and thus a fourth measure – the number of frequency components (number of peaks) – has been used. The method has been described in detail elsewhere [*Cumberbatch* et al., 1980].

Statistics. When correlated samples were analysed the Wilcoxon matched-pair rank sign test was used and when separate samples were compared the Mann-Whitney U test was used. Relationships were sought by means of the linear correlation coefficient.

Results

Correlation with Age. In the largest series, the series of depressed patients, n = 40, significant negative correlations were found between age and the delta activity in all leads, the theta activity in all leads on the left side and at C4 and

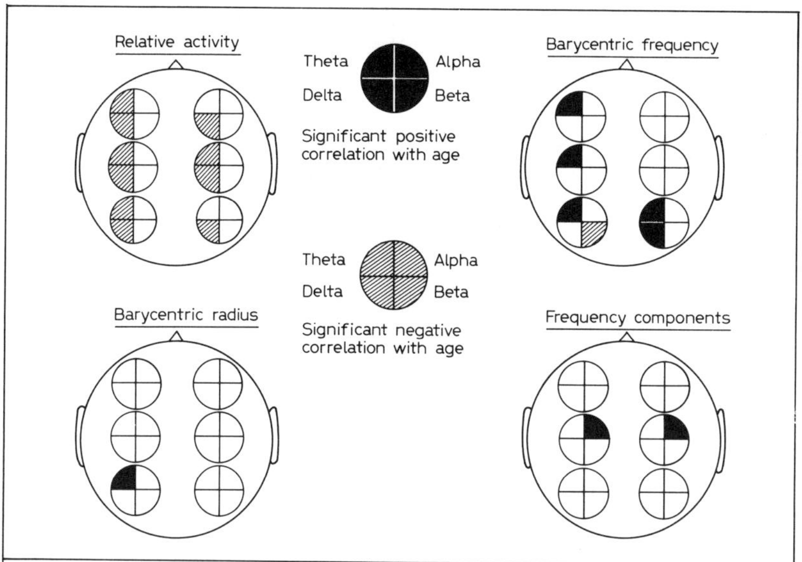

1

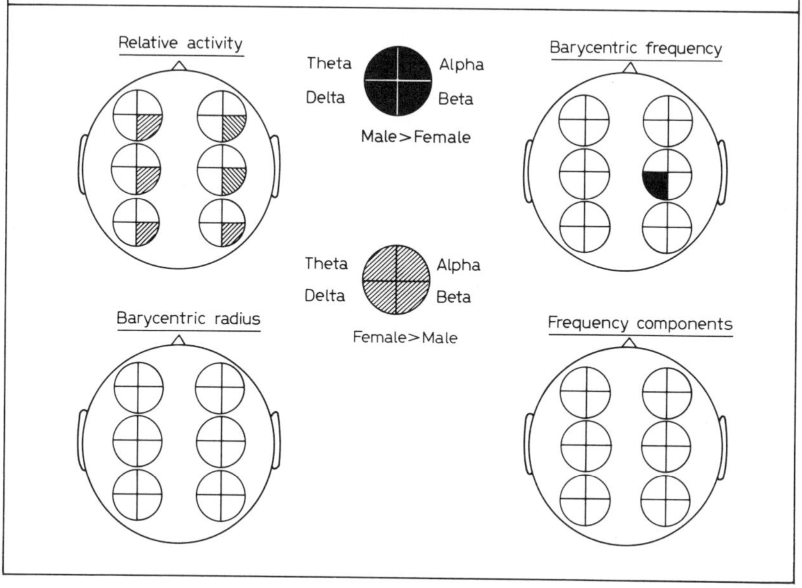

2

Fig. 1. Correlations between age and geometrical spectral descriptors of the EEG. Linear correlation coefficient. Correlation indicated if significant at the 5% level. Depressed patients, n = 40.

Fig. 2. Differences in geometrical spectral descriptors of the EEG between male, n = 16, and female, n = 24, depressed patients, n = 40. Mann-Whitney U test. Differences indicated if significant at the 5% level.

the beta frequency at 01. Significant positive correlations were found with the theta frequency in all leads on the left side and at 02, the theta radius at 01 and the number of frequency components in alpha in the central leads (fig. 1).

Sex Differences. In the series of depressed patients, n = 40, women were found to have significantly higher beta activity in all leads while the male patients had significantly higher delta frequency at C4 (fig. 2).

Drug-Free Patients versus Patients who had had Minor and Irregular Doses of Tricyclics of Minor Tranquilizers during the Last Week. In this comparison only few significant differences occurred. The completely drug-free patients had significantly lower beta frequency at 01 and significantly higher theta radius at F3 but all other differences were non-significant (fig. 3).

Healthy Volunteers versus Depressed Patients. The healthy volunteers were found to have significantly higher delta and theta activity in all leads except 01 as well as a larger number of frequency components in theta at C3 and 01, while the depressed patients had higher theta frequency at C4 and 02 and more frequency components in beta at F4 (fig. 4).

Psychotic versus Non-Psychotic Depressed Patients. Only few significant differences emerged between the 19 psychotic depressed patients and the 21 non-psychotic depressed patients. The non-psychotic patients had higher beta frequency in the occipital leads and more frequency components in beta at 02 (fig. 5).

Interhemispheric Differences in Healthy Volunteers and Depressed Patients. In the group of healthy volunteers, n = 20, delta and theta activity was found to be significantly higher on the right side in the central and occipital leads while the alpha and beta activity was found to be significantly higher on the left side in the corresponding leads. The delta frequency was higher on the left side in the central leads and the theta frequency was higher on left side in both central and occipital leads (fig. 6). In depressed patients a reversed pattern was found. The delta and theta activity was now significantly higher on the left side in the central leads while the alpha activity was significantly higher on the right side. Also as concerns the frequency measures, a reversed pattern was found in the central leads with higher delta and theta frequency on the right side (fig. 7).

The results concerning interhemispheric differences are summarized in figure 8. As can be seen the most pronounced differences between healthy volunteers and depressed patients occur in the central leads where an interhemispheric shift is found in both activity and frequency measures.

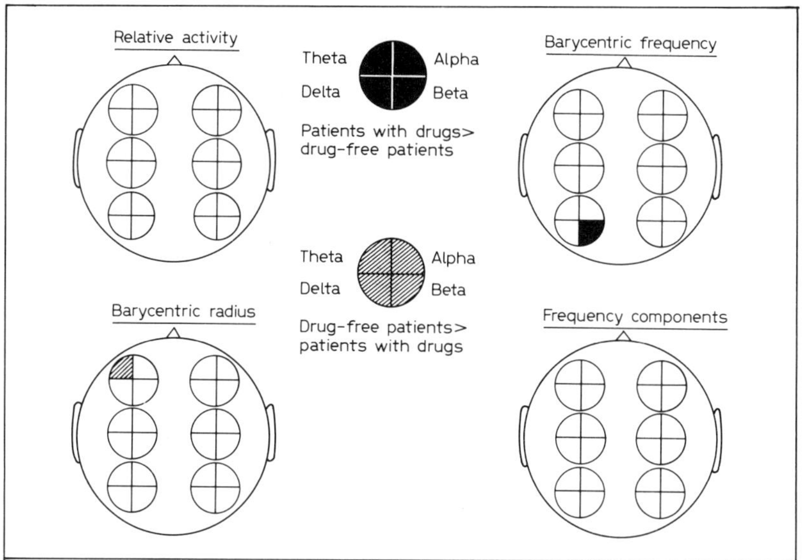

3

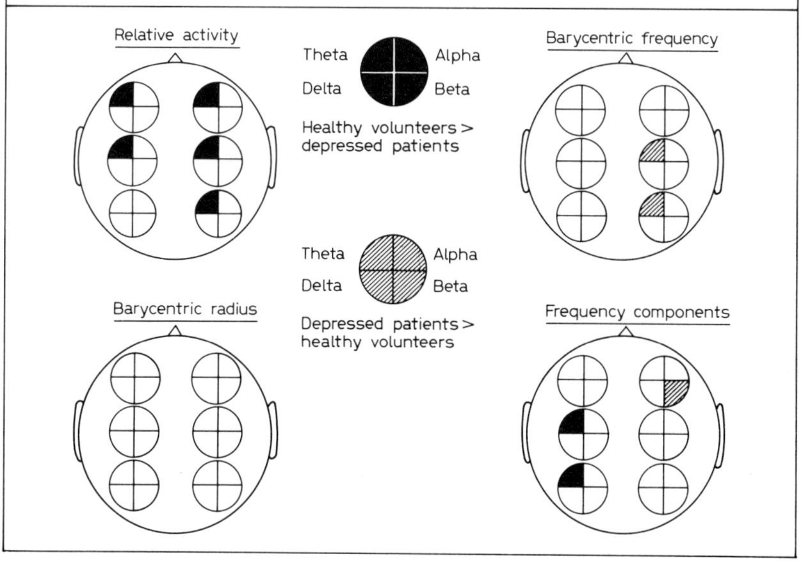

4

Fig. 3. Differences in geometrical spectral descriptors of the EEG between patients who had minor doses of tricyclics or minor tranquilizers during the last week, n = 22, and completely drug-free patients, n = 18. Depressed patients, n = 40. Differences indicated if significant at the 5% level. Mann-Whitney U test.

Fig. 4. Differences in geometrical spectral descriptors of the EEG between healthy volunteers, n = 20, and depressed patients, n = 40, comparable for age and sex. Differences indicated if significant at the 5% level. Mann-Whitney U test.

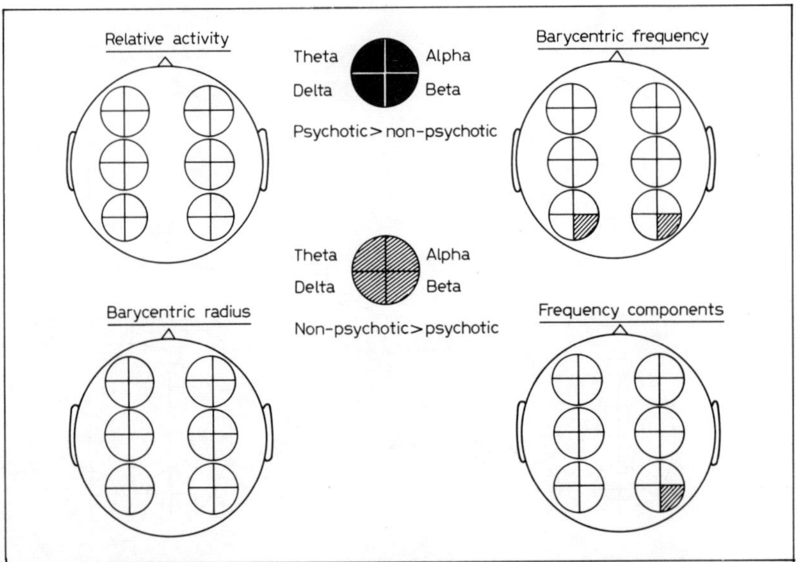

5

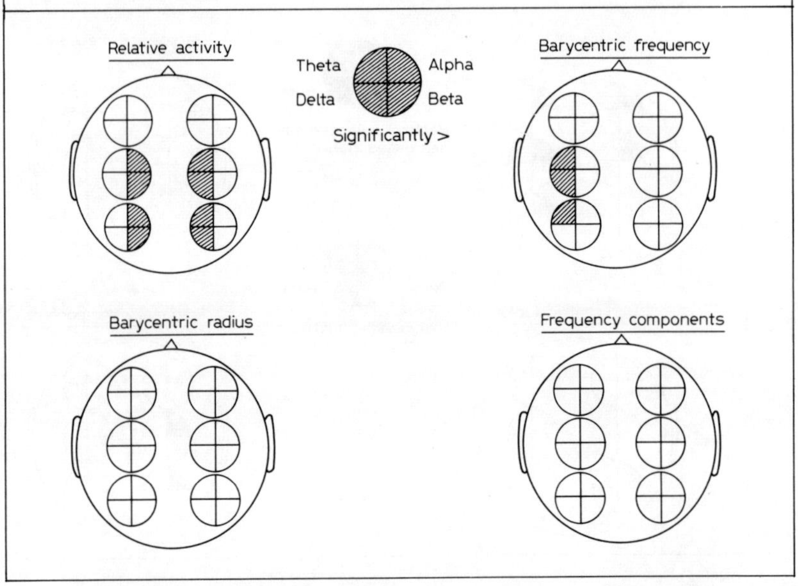

6

Fig. 5. Differences in geometrical spectral descriptors of the EEG between psychotic, n = 19, and non-psychotic, n = 21, depressed patients, n = 40. Differences indicated if significant at the 5% level. Mann-Whitney U test.

Fig. 6. Interhemispheric differences in geometrical spectral descriptors of the EEG in healthy volunteers, n = 20. Differences indicated if significant at the 5% level. Wilcoxon matched pair rank sign test.

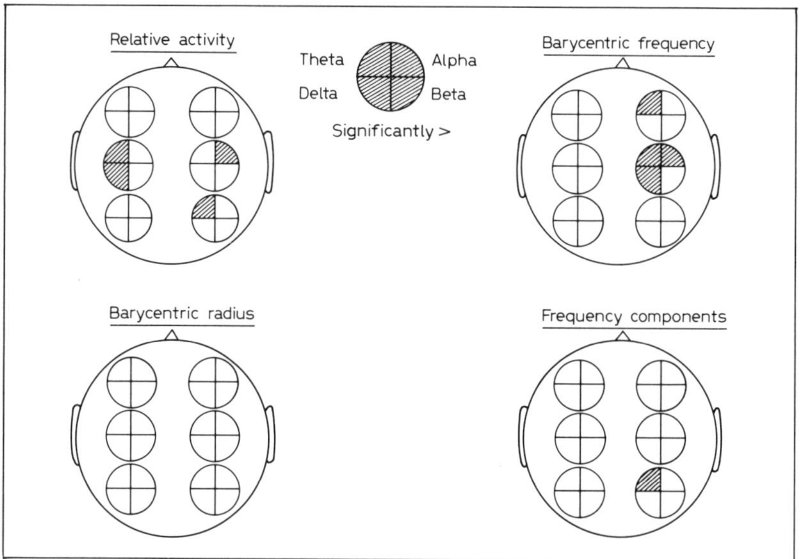

7

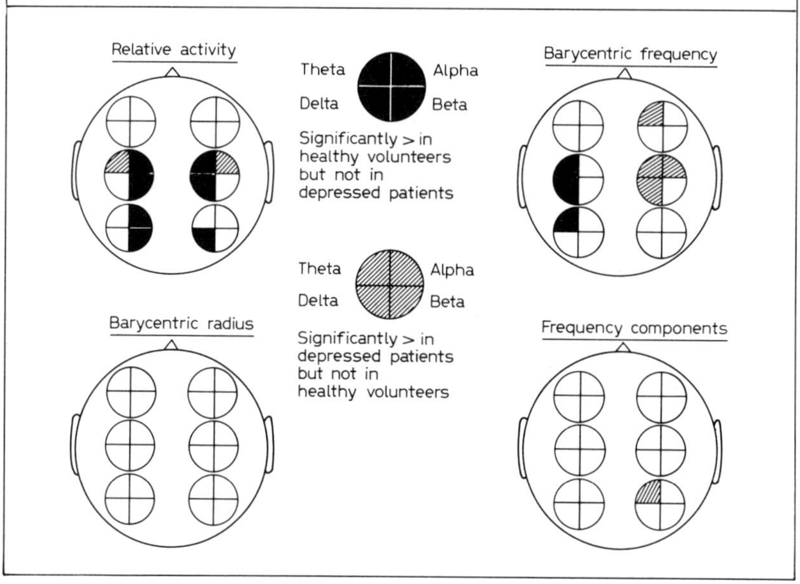

8

Fig. 7. Interhemispheric differences in geometrical spectral descriptors of the EEG in depressed patients, n = 40. Differences indicated if significant at the 5% level. Wilcoxon matched pair rank sign test.

Fig. 8. A comparison between interhemispheric differences present in healthy volunteers, n = 20, and in depressed patients, n = 40. An interhemispheric difference is considered if significant at the 5% level. Wilcoxon matched pair rank sign test.

Discussion

The age correlations found are most pronounced in the delta and theta frequency bands but occasional correlations also occur in the alpha and beta frequency bands. The sex differences are most pronounced in the beta activity and is in line with earlier results [*Flor-Henry and Koles,* 1980]. In summary the age correlations and the sex differences are so pronounced that it seems important to use carefully age- and sex-matched series when comparisons are sought, or at least to include some correction for these variables.

The question about drugs is always extremely important in clinical research. It is always best to use completely drug-free patients, but sometimes when newly admitted patients are investigated it is impossible to control the drug intake the week prior to admission. In this situation it is also impossible to rely completely on the information given by the patient as occasional doses are easily forgotten. Regular use of therapeutic doses of psychoactive drugs give pronounced differences in the EEG measures [*Itil,* 1974; *Saletu* et al., 1980]. However, the importance of small and irregular doses is not clear and, according to the results in the present study, this influence seems to be of minor importance.

When healthy volunteers and depressed patients of comparable age and with the same sex distribution are compared, the most pronounced differences are lower activity in all leads in the lower frequency bands in the depressed patients. The results seem to be in line with earlier results [for a review, see *Perris,* 1980]. When depressed patients with psychotic and non-psychotic depressive syndromes are compared, only few significant differences occur. However, this lack of differences is not surprising. According to the ratings by means of CPRS no significant difference exist in total rating score between these groups, and our earlier studies have shown that differences in symptomatology are much more important than differences in diagnostic category [*Monakhov* et al., 1979].

As concerns interhemispheric differences a reversed pattern is found in depressed patients as compared to healthy volunteers. In healthy volunteers the delta and theta activity is significantly higher on the right side while alpha and beta activity is higher on the left side. In depressed patients the pattern is reversed. The differences are most pronounced in the central leads. Also in the delta and theta frequency there is a complete reversal of dominance in the central leads. The results are in line with earlier results by means of MIA where lower amplitudes were found on the left side during depression, especially in the alpha frequency band [*d'Elia and Perris,* 1974; *Perris,* 1980].

In conclusion the geometrical spectral descriptors of the EEG seem to give promising results, and it is very interesting that the differences found are in line with results obtained by means of other methods of EEG analysis. This consistency indicates that the still unknown phenomena beyond the results obtained are robust and consistent, not depending on special characteristics of the method used.

Summary

Healthy volunteers of comparable age and sex have been compared to depressed patients by means of geometrical spectral descriptors of the EEG. A further measure of the variability of the amplitude – the number of frequency components – has also been used. The age correlations and sex differences seem to be so important that it is concluded that groups that will be compared should be matched for age and sex or a correction for these variables should be made. Small and irregular doses of tricyclics of minor tranquilizers used during the week prior to the EEG examination seem to be of minor importance. The division in psychotic and non-psychotic depressive syndromes give only few significant differences in geometrical spectral descriptors of the EEG, and it is suggested that the symptomatology as determined by means of clinical rating is of more importance than clinical diagnosis. Interhemispheric differences found in healthy volunteers are found to be reversed in depressed patients, in line with earlier results.

References

Asberg, M.; Perris, C.; Schalling, D.; Sedvall, G.: CPRS – the development and application of a psychiatric rating scale. Acta psychiat. scand. suppl. *271* (1978).

Cumberbatch, J.; Knorring, L. von; Perris, C.: Some methodological aspects concerning geometrical spectral descriptors of the computerised EEG. Proc. 2nd Symp. on Clinical Neurophysiological Aspects of Psychopathological Conditions, Capri 1980.

d'Elia, G.: Unilateral electroconvulsive therapy. Acta psychiat. scand. suppl. *215* (1970).

d'Elia, G.; Knorring, L. von; Perris, C.: Non-psychotic depressive disorders, a ten year follow up. Acta psychiat. scand. suppl. *255:* 173–186 (1974).

d'Elia, G.; Perris, C.: Cerebral functional dominance and memory functions. Acta psychiat. scand. *255:* suppl., pp. 143–157 (1974).

Flor-Henry, P.; Koles, Z.J.: EEG studies in depression, mania and normals: evidence for partial shifts in the affective psychosis. Adv. biol. Psychiat., vol. 4, pp. 21–43 (Karger, Basel 1980).

Itil, T.M.: Quantitative pharmaco-electroencephalography. Mod. Probl. Pharmacopsychiat., vol. 8, pp. 43–75 (Karger, Basel 1974).

Kemali, D.; Vacca, L.; Nolfe, G.; Iorio, G.; De Carlo, R.: Hemispheric EEG quantitative asymmetries in schizophrenics and depressed patients. Adv. biol. Psychiat., vol. 4, 14–20 (Karger, Basel 1980).

Marciano, F.; Nolfe, G.: Geometrical spectral descriptors. Internal report No. 7 (Institute of Cybernetics, National Council of Research, Naples 1977).

Monakhov, K.; Perris, C.; Botskarev, V.; Knorring, L. von; Nikiforov, A.: Functional interhemispheric differences in relation to various psychopathological components of the depressive syndromes. Neuropsychobiology *5:* 143–155 (1979).

Perris, C.: A study of bipolar (manic-depressive) and unipolar recurrent depressive psychoses. Acta psychiat. scand. suppl. *194* (1966).

Perris, C.: Central measures of depression; in van Prag, Handbook of biol. psychiat. (Dekker, New York 1980).

Saletu, B.; Grunberger, J.; Linzmayer, L.; Anderer, P.: Classification and assessment of pharmacodynamics of SGD-SCHA 1059 (Binodaline) by quantitative EEG and psychometric analyses. Adv. biol. Psychiat., vol. 4, pp. 140–166 (Karger, Basel 1980).

C. Perris, MD, Department of Psychiatry, University of Umeå, S-90185 Umeå (Sweden)

Adv. biol. Psychiat., vol. 6, pp. 50–53 (Karger, Basel 1981)

Neurophysiology of Mentality

N.P. Bechtereva, S.V. Medvedev

Institute for Experimental Medicine of the USSR Academy of Medical Science, Leningrad, USSR

Investigation into the cerebral maintenance of mental activity involves study of at least two main questions: (1) Where exactly in the brain are those areas which take part in the maintenance of this function. (2) What exactly occurs in these areas thus reflecting (determining) (a) the conditions for proceeding mental activity, and (b) the proceeding of the activity per se?

(1) An answer to the first question historically stemmed first from the so-called clinical-anatomical parallels considerably corroborated by the modern neuropsychology. From the 1930s, data on cerebral structural organization of the maintenance of mental activity started to accumulate owing to pointed electric stimulations of the cortex [*Penfield,* 1958; *Ojemann,* 1979] and somewhat later of the subcortical brain structures. Practical application of the indwelling electrode technique enriched the possibilities of obtaining this kind of data and determined the possibility and, sometimes, the necessity of additional examinations of some cerebral physiological processes during performance of various physiological tests. Performance of the studies under different ambient conditions for the organism and inner conditions for the brain revealed that the reproducibility of the dynamics of physiological parameters proves stable in but a few structures which were there upon determined as the rigid links of the system for mental activity maintenance. In other areas, the reproducible dynamics of physiological processes might appear depending on the conditions for the activity development [the flexible links of the system; *Bechtereva,* 1966].

The data on principles and concrete forms of the structural-functional system for mental functions maintenance made it possible to commence study of the second main question: What exactly occurs during development of mental activity in those brain areas which take part in the maintenance of mental activity?

(2a) Study of those physiological parameters had been undertaken which characterized the readjustment of functioning level in different brain areas involved in mental activity. The study revealed that, although practically all the physiological processes can be used to that purpose, the most adequate processes for studying the slowly occurring readjustments of the brain state were slow electric events different in their intensity.

(2b) Investigation into the subtle readjustments related to the character of activity per se can be most adequately performed with the aid of readjustments in the impulse activity of neuronal populations.

Studies of the impulse activity of neuronal populations in the cortex and in subcortical structures of the thalamus, striopallidar system, medio-basal portions of the temporal lobes, upper portions of the brain stem, and other cerebral structures during perception and uttering of words, or during more complex mental activity, have shown that readjustments related to the character of activity can develop locally, in the 'active' areas of these structures. These readjustments (patterns) are characterized by changes in the frequency and structure of the impulse flow the latter, apparently, being closely related to readjustments of interaction among neurons within the population or, rather, the working ensemble of neurons. The local processes in different brain areas involved in the maintenance of mental processes are dynamically interrelated, the closeness of connection among different areas being dependent on phases of mental activity. The evolved apparatus for mathematical-technical analysis of local as well as systemic processes made it possible to single out of the patterns of local impulse activity of neuronal populations, and of interaction among different brain areas, the signs of semantic differentiation of semantic groups and to predict the result of decision-making. Analysis of the local patterns revealed the 'short-lived' readjustments in the structure of impulse flow characterized by the appearance of functionally significant grouped sequences of discharges with three or more quite certain intervals. The pattern consisted of an aggregate of such grouped sequences of discharges.

More stable local neurophysiological correlates of mental processes were found in the form of grouped sequences of discharges, the significant factor of which involved not the absolute values of intervals between discharges but the correlation in length of successive intervals [*Bundzen and David,* 1979]. In this way the sequences of discharges were singled out comprising at least 6 intervals whose 'span of life' (i.e. reproducibility in analogous conditions) was considerably longer (days, weeks).

Psychological tests for decision-making have revealed that the significant factor underlying the prediction of the decision-making results involves the interaction among certain brain areas.

Significance of the factor of interaction among different brain areas for maintenance of mental activity is determined by the distributed rather than local, systemic maintenance (coding) of mental processes.

The question of the mechanism of interaction has particularly urgently risen when studying the activity of the system for mental activity maintenance where it is very important to consider the number of links with relatively major local readjustments occurring in them; at the same time, the factor of dynamic interaction among different areas turned out to be extremely significant. Consequently, a study of the cerebral conditions for the interaction has been undertaken as one of elements of the complex thorough investigation of its mechanisms. The impedance study had been carried out in a peculiar clinical model in which a frequency-selective artificial stable functional connection [applied usually to therapy of parkinsonism; *Smirnov,* 1976] was established between two brain areas with the aid of a simultaneous electric stimulation. This connection further proved able to reveal itself at the light stimulation of the same frequency, too. In the recordings of the impedance between two brain areas, a drop of impedance by 95% occurred at the moment of reaching the 'active' frequency during trying different frequencies of the light stimulation. In the course of mental activity, short and less significant drops of impedance occurred between the two involved areas, the impedance gradually diminishing afterwards. These data indicate the possibility of temporal occurrence in the brain of the channels with increased conductivity facilitating the conditions of interaction among different brain areas. The further most important aspect of this question involves investigation of what exactly is being transmitted over these channels of increased conductivity.

Summary

Cerebral structural-functional maintenance of mental activity is sustained by a cortical-subcortical system with links of different grades of rigidity. The possibility of participation of cerebral areas in this maintenance is determined by their functional state, the most adequate parameter of the latter involving the slow electric processes. Physiological correlates of the activity per se involve the local rearrangements of the impulse activity frequencies and structure as well as the interaction among the involved cerebral areas. Dynamic formation of channels with increased conductivity within the brain is supposed to be one of the conditions for this interaction.

References

Bechtereva, N.P.: Nekotorye principialnye voprocy izutchenia neirofiziologitcheskich osnov psichitcheskich iavleni tcheloveka. In: Glubokie struktury golovnogo mozga tcheloveka v norme i patologii, pp. 18–21 (Publ. 'Nauka', Moscow 1966).

Bundzen, P.V.; David, E.: O roli kogerencii neironnoi aktivnosti v kodirovanii i dekodirovanni informacii. Hum. Physiol. *5:* 3–13 (1979).

Ojemann, G.A.: Individual variability in cortical localization of language. J. Neurosurg. *50:* 164–169 (1979).

Penfield, W.: The role of the temporal cortex in recall of past. Experience and interpretation of the present. Ciba Fdn Symp. on Neurological Basis of Behaviour, London 1958, pp. 149–172.

Smirnov, V.M.: Stereotaxitcheskaia nevrologia (Publ. 'Medicina', Leningrad 1976).

N.P. Bechtereva, MD, Institute for Experimental Medicine,
Pavlov's Street, 12, 197022 Leningrad (USSR)

Adv. biol. Psychiat., vol. 6, pp. 54–59 (Karger, Basel 1981)

Altered Brain Functional Organisation in Psychosis: Brain-Behaviour Relationships

John H. Gruzelier, John F. Connolly, Steven R. Hirsch
Department of Psychiatry, Charing Cross Hospital Medical School, London, England

After a decade of intensive research in cerebral lateralisation and psychopathology [*Gruzelier and Flor-Henry,* 1979; *Gruzelier,* 1981] one of the research strategies necessary to elucidate the matter further is to seek relationships between the neurophysiological or neuropsychological measures on the one hand, and the reported symptoms, behavioural signs and syndromes on the other. Because there is growing disenchantment [*Kety,* 1980] with conventional diagnostic practices, research in psychopathology may be on a safer wicket if groups are defined on the basis of symptoms, signs and syndromes, though even here reliability is less than desired. Therefore, the ultimate goal of the psychopathologist to find objective measures of function is of utmost importance.

Electrodermal Activity

Recordings of bilateral electrodermal responses have until recently shown an asymmetry consistent in one direction in schizophrenia and the opposite asymmetry in some cases of depression [*Gruzelier,* 1979]. A recent investigation where inconsistent results were found [*Gruzelier* et al., 1981a] involved patients entering a drug study in which florid symptoms were one criterion for entry and another was a diagnosis of schizophrenia on the Catego system [*Wing* et al., 1974]. In this system diagnosis is based on a hierarchy which places emphasis on certain characteristic symptoms, for example Schneiderian first-rank symptoms in the case of nuclear schizophrenia, rather than the overall balance of symptoms, such that the coexistence of Schneiderian symptoms and mania would lead to a diagnosis of schizophrenia and when manic symptoms coexisted with a predominantly depressive picture the diagnosis would be mania. We gained the impression that many cases with the discrepant electrodermal asymmetry had manic symptoms and might be diagnosed differently by another method. We set out to relate the direction of the lateral asymmetry to the 38 Catego syndromes and 19 items of the Brief Psychiatric Rating Scale (BPRS) [*Overall and Gorham,* 1962].

The results obtained on the 23 trial patients with psychophysiology were reexamined with the next 25 consecutive admissions for schizophrenia with a Catego diagnosis and an electrodermal response asymmetry [*Gruzelier and Manchanda,* 1981]. This afforded a replication and the present report is confined to an analysis of the total sample of 48 patients. They consisted of 30 men and 18 women, none of whom had received neuroleptics for at least 3 weeks and virtually all were tested within 4 days of admission. Their ages ranged from 18 to 68 years. Numbers of hospital admissions ranged from 1 to 24. Methods of electrodermal measurement have been described elsewhere [*Gruzelier* et al., 1981b]. Responses were examined to 15, 90 dB, 5 s, 1,000-Hz tones with controlled rise and decay times. We found that the majority of recent admissions who were non-responsive to moderate intensity 70-dB tones responded at the louder intensity. 29 patients had larger right-hand skin conductance responses (R > L) and 19 had larger left-hand responses (L > R). The psychiatric evaluations were on the same day, or the day before or after testing.

Syndromes and ratings in which there were significant differences either in magnitude or in the number of patients identified were as follows. Those with larger left-hand responses had more pressure of speech and grandiosity on the BPRS, while on the PSE they had more simple ideas of reference, hypomania, situational anxiety, delusions of grandeur, hypochondriasis, and depressive delusions and hallucinations. Those patients with larger right-hand responses had on the BPRS more emotional withdrawal, motor retardation, blunted affect and uncooperativeness, while on the PSE they were more reticent in interview, were more irritable with the interviewer, had more slowness and simple depression. Thus, there appeared a bipolarity colouring self-concepts, speech, cognition, affect and movement with L > R patients showing high arousal and R > L patients low arousal. Schneiderian symptoms did not distinguish them. Beyond this the R > L patients were seen as lacking in sociability.

These distinguishing features were submitted to a principal components factor analysis and in order to describe the factors accurately the particular items contributing to the syndromes of the present patients were examined. The first factor (table I) contributed almost twice the variance of the second factor. Its bipolarity aptly described the two groups, one at each pole. The factor structure was then simplified with a varimax rotation, also shown in table I. Of the six main factors three characterised the florid group: heightened arousal, exaggerated self-awareness and exaggerated bodily concern, and three characterised the non-florid group: slowness and emotional withdrawal, simple depression, and social withdrawal. In order to obtain the most economical set of discriminating variables ignoring items which, while differentiating the groups correlated highly with a better discriminant, stepwise discriminant function analyses were carried

Table I. The principal factor (iterative method) and six sprincipal factors after varimax rotation [*Kim*, 1970]

Factor label and % of variance	Main items and loadings
1 Florid – non-florid (L > R – R > L) 23.8 %	situational anxiety, phobias, anxiety avoidance (–0.53); hypomanic affect and speech, euphoria, ideomotor pressure, grandiose ideas (–0.49) depressive hallucinations, delusions guilt, catastrophe, hypochondriasis (–0.45) religious delusions and of grandiose ability and identity (–0.45) grandiosity: exaggerated opinion of self and abilities (–0.42) simple ideas of reference (self consciousness) (–0.37) pressure of speech (–0.37) emotional withdrawal: no contact with interviewer (0.68) blunted affect: reduced emotional tone (0.65) slowness: slow speech, movements, restricted quantity of speech, muteness (0.65) motor retardation: reduced energy level, slowed movements (0.60) reticent and unforthcoming in interview (0.50)
1 Slowness, emotional withdrawal 37.9 %	slowness (0.73), motor retardation (0.70), emotional withdrawal (0.66), reticence (0.60), uncooperativeness (0.53), blunted affect (0.49)
2 Heightened arousal 18.3 %	Situational anxiety (0.82), hypomania (0.62), religious and grandiose delusions (0.62), pressure of speech (0.51)
3 Exaggerated self-awareness 15.3 %	grandiosity (0.86), ideas of reference (0.65)
4 Exaggerated bodily concern and depressive delusions 13.1 %	hypochondriasis (0.94), depressive delusions (0.46)
5 Simple depression 9.8 %	simple depression (0.90)
6 Social withdrawal 5.7 %	blunted affect (0.63), emotional withdrawal (0.51). social unease: social withdrawal, lack of selfconfidence (0.42)

out. Eight variables classified 46/48 patients. The profiles of the two groups were enlarged to include *conceptual disorganisation, self-neglect and worrying* in the case of R > L patients and *unusual thought content, somatic concern, and mannerisms and posturing* in the case of L > R patients.

There is a striking resemblance between the profile of the R > L patients and the classical description of schizophrenia by *Kraepelin* and *Bleuler* with its interpersonal disturbance, lack of affect and motivation, and thought disorder. On the other hand, the florid psychotic features which characterised the L > R patients are characteristic of a manic or schizo-affective psychosis. It is noteworthy that in both groups Schneiderian symptoms were found, which *Kety* [1980] notes are 'neither characteristic nor discriminating' and claims that 'the acute psychoses in which they are often found do not have the type of onset or course, the family history, the fundamental symptoms, prognosis or response to treatment that are associated with schizophrenia'. The move away from the classical view was in part because of poor reliability in evaluating the symptoms. A biological correlate of the syndrome may therefore have a practical application.

Cortical-Evoked Responses

We examined the phenomenon of saturation whereby instead of increasing monotonically with stimulus intensity the amplitude of the EP levels off or declines [*Hillyard* et al., 1978]. This may reflect a cortical modulation of input akin to the phenomenon of augmenting-reducing [*Buchsbaum and Pfefferbaum,* 1971], though a direct analogy is not intended [*Connolly and Gruzelier,* 1981].

Bilateral recordings were obtained from temporal (T3, and T4) and occipital (01, 02) placements in addition to vertex and were referred to linked ears [*Connolly and Gruzelier,* 1981]. The patients fulfilled the Catego criteria for schizophrenia. They were 11 men and 5 women, all recent admissions and free of neuroleptics for at least 3 weeks.

In support of a left hemisphere model of schizophrenia patients differed from controls at the left temporal site; some showing less saturation in the amplitude of the P100 peak. In fact 6/16 (37.5%) displayed this compared with 1/22 (4.5%) controls (Fisher's test, $p < 0.03$ one-tailed). There was also a group difference in hemispheric asymmetry in the N120 peak at occipital sites; patients showed less saturation on the left and controls less saturation on the right (Fisher's test, $p < 0.05$). This effect applied to only 4/16 patients and 5/22 controls. There was no correspondence between the patients showing the effect at the two sites. Finally, patients were distinguished from controls by a lateral asymmetry in the direction of lower P100–N120 amplitudes on the left side ($F = 4.08$, d.f. = 1.34, $p < 0.05$).

The fact that only about a third of patients showed an EP asymmetry at each bilateral placement, yet all showed an electrodermal response asymmetry and a left hemisphere deficit on a tachistoscopic task [*Connolly* et al., 1979] implies that the EP measure here is relatively insensitive. Perhaps the role of electrocortical recording from surface electrodes lies in providing evidence of asymmetries in dynamic processes, or in levels of processing with which to supplement behavioural tasks.

The small numbers involved make these results of exploratory interest. Nevertheless, their potential relevance is suggested by a difference in the Catego syndromes of the 6 patients showing no saturation in the left temporal P100 when compared with the remaining 10 patients. The former had higher scores on nuclear schizophrenia ($F = 7.08$, d.f. = 1.14, $p < 0.05$). Those not showing saturation at the left occipital site had higher scores on situational anxiety ($F = 5.24$, d.f. = 1.13, $p < 0.05$) and hypomania ($F = 6.36$, d.f. = 1.13, $p < 0.05$).

Working Model

The model with which the electrodermal, electrocortical and behavioural evidence is integrated is currently as follows. Schizophrenia and psychoses with a manic component involve a left temporal disorder. Evidence for this is reviewed elsewhere [*Gruzelier,* 1981] and includes evidence of a left visual field deficit in processing lexical stimuli in both schizophrenia and mania and the coincidence of Schneiderian symptoms with less saturation of the P100 peak at the left temporal site. However, the bidirectional asymmetries in the electrodermal-orienting response suggests that the pattern of temporal-limbic activation differs in the classical schizophrenia syndrome of *Kraepelin* and *Bleuler* from the florid syndrome with hypomanic overtones. Classical schizophrenia with its retarded motility, impoverished speech and sometimes muteness involves reduced left hemisphere activation. The florid psychotic syndrome with its pressure of speech and flight of ideas involves enhanced left hemisphere activation. The left hemisphere disturbance alters the balance of activity of both hemispheres because (1) their functions are integrated and (2) there is evidence of reciprocal interactions between them in the control of arousal [*Gruzelier* et al., 1981]. A disturbance of brain functional organisation ensues with an over-reliance on the left hemisphere in the florid syndrome and on the right hemisphere in the classical syndrome.

References

Buchsbaum, M.; Pfefferbaum, A.: Individual differences in stimulus intensity response. Psychophysiology *8:* 600–611 (1971).

Connolly, J.F.; Gruzelier, J.H.; Kleinman, K.M.; Hirsch, S.R.: Lateralised abnormalities in hemisphere-specific tachistoscopic tasks in psychiatric patients and controls; in Gruzelier, Flor-Henry, Hemisphere asymmetries of function in psychopathology (Elsevier, Amsterdam 1979).

Connolly, J.F.; Gruzelier, J.H.: Amplitude and latency changes in the visual evoked potential (VEP) to different stimulus intensities. Psychology (in press, 1981).

Gruzelier, J.H.: Lateral asymmetries in electrodermal activity and psychosis; in Gruzelier, Flor-Henry, Hemisphere asymmetries of function in psychopathology (Elsevier, Amsterdam 1979).

Gruzelier, J.H.: Cerebral laterality and psychopathology: fact and fiction (editorial). Psychol. Med. *11:* 1–9 (1981).

Gruzelier, J.H.; Manchanda, R.: The syndrome of schizophrenia: lateral asymmetries in electrodermal responses (in preparation, 1981).

Gruzelier, J.H.; Connolly, J.F.; Eves, F.F.; Hirsch, S.R.; Zaki, S.A.; Weller, M.P.I.; Yorkston, N.J.: Effect of propranolol and phenothiazines on electrodermal orienting and habituation in schizophrenia. Psychol. Med. *11:* 93–108 (1981).

Gruzelier, J.H.; Eves, F.F.; Connolly, J.F.: Reciprocal hemispheric influences on response habituation in the electrodermal system. Physiological Psychology (in press, 1981a).

Gruzelier, J.H.; Flor-Henry, P.H.: Hemisphere asymmetries of function in psychopathology (Elsevier, Amsterdam 1979).

Hillyard, S.A.; Picton, T.W.; Regan, D.: Sensation, perception and attention: analysis using ERPs; in Callaway, Tueting, Koslow, Event-related brain potentials in man (Academic Press, New York 1978).

Kety, S.S.: The syndrome of schizophrenia: unresolved questions and opportunities for research. Br. J. Psychiat. *136:* 421–436 (1980).

Overall, J.E.; Gorham, D.R.: The brief psychiatric rating scale. Psychol. Rep. *10:* 799–812 (1962).

Wing, J.K.; Cooper, J.E.; Sartorius, N.: Measurement and classification of psychiatric symptoms (Cambridge University Press, London 1974).

J.H. Gruzelier, PhD, Department of Psychiatry, Charing, Cross Hospital Medical School, Fulham Palace Road, London W6 8RF (England)

Adv. biol. Psychiat., vol. 6, pp. 60–67 (Karger, Basel 1981)

Studies in Right/Left Hemispheric Energy Oscillations in Schizophrenia, Mania, Depression and Normals

P. Flor-Henry, Z.J. Koles

University of Alberta, Alberta Hospital, Edmonton, Alta., Canada

Many investigations in the last 10 years have shown that the endogenous psychoses are related to complex alterations in the organization of cerebral laterality [1–4]. At the same time, some workers [5, 6] have suggested that abnormal interhemispheric relationships also represent perhaps a fundamental aspect of psychosis. As a contribution to the question of interhemispheric organization in psychosis the present authors investigated the oscillations through time of right/left hemispheric energy in 22 normals, 19 schizophrenics, 20 depressives and 21 manic patients, all of whom were unmedicated.

Methods

An EEG from each of the subject, amplified by a Grass electroencephalograph, was recorded during a 3-min epoch in the following conditions: rest, eyes open, eyes closed, and during verbal and spatial cognitive activation. Only the resting situations (eyen open, eyes closed) are reported here. The EEG signal was analyzed off-line and after digital conversion at 120 points/s was fast Fourier transformed in segments of 32 points (Hewlett-Packard 1200 S minicomputer). Successive segments were obtained by shifting 8 points, thus giving an effective sampling rate of 120/8 = 15 points/s (fig. 1). These were analyzed after power component separation into 8–13, 13–20 and 20–50 Hz bands. The average power ratios over the 3 min were calculated $\log_e (\bar{P}_r/\bar{P}_l) \rightarrow \log_e \bar{P}$ and $\log_e (\bar{T}_r/\bar{T}_l) \rightarrow \log_e \bar{T}$ (fig. 2) (from P_3, P_4 and T_3, T_4 of the international 10–20 system, against vertex reference C_z). At each sampling interval (i.e. 15 times/s) $\log_e (P_r/P_l) \rightarrow \log_e P$ and $\log_e (T_r/T_l) \rightarrow \log_e T$ were subtracted from the combined average giving $\log_e (P/\bar{P})$, $\log_e (T/T)$ (fig. 3) and thereby a measure of right/left hemispheric energy oscillations through time (fig. 4). The number of right/left shifts per second for the three frequency bands were calculated (t test, all probabilities $p < 0.025$ or $p < 0.05$) as well as the number of intervals present which were shorter than 0.07 and 0.35 s and greater than 0.60 s. This was done for the temporal and parietal regions.

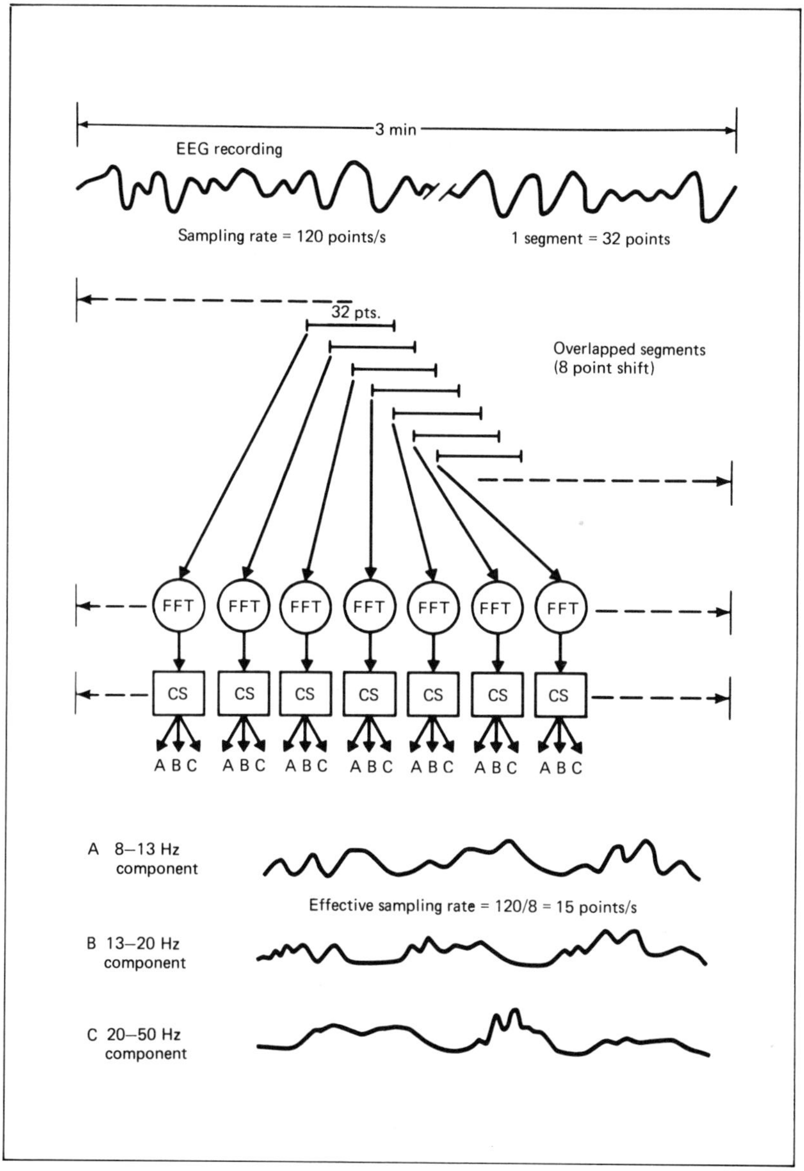

Fig. 1. Sketch of technique of power spectral analysis. FFT = Fast Fourier transform; CS = power component separation.

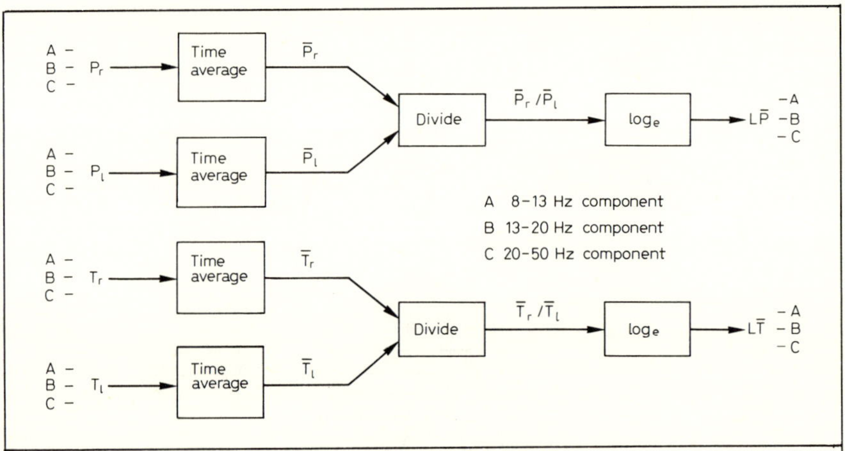
A – B – P_r
Time average
$\bar{P}_r$
A – B – C – P_l
Time average
$\bar{P}_l$
Divide
$\bar{P}_r / \bar{P}_l$
$\log_e$
$L\bar{P}$ –A –B –C
A 8–13 Hz component
B 13–20 Hz component
C 20–50 Hz component
A – B – C – T_r
Time average
$\bar{T}_r$
A – B – C – T_l
Time average
$\bar{T}_l$
Divide
$\bar{T}_r / \bar{T}_l$
$\log_e$
$L\bar{T}$ –A –B –C

2

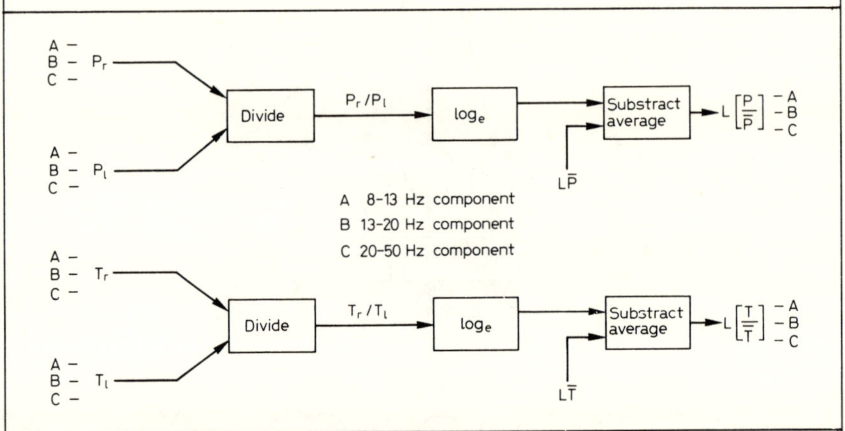
A – B – C – P_r
A – B – C – P_l
Divide
P_r / P_l
$\log_e$
Substract average
$L\bar{P}$
$L\left[\frac{P}{\bar{P}}\right]$ –A –B –C
A 8-13 Hz component
B 13-20 Hz component
C 20-50 Hz component
A – B – C – T_r
A – B – C – T_l
Divide
T_r / T_l
$\log_e$
Substract average
$L\bar{T}$
$L\left[\frac{T}{\bar{T}}\right]$ –A –B –C

3

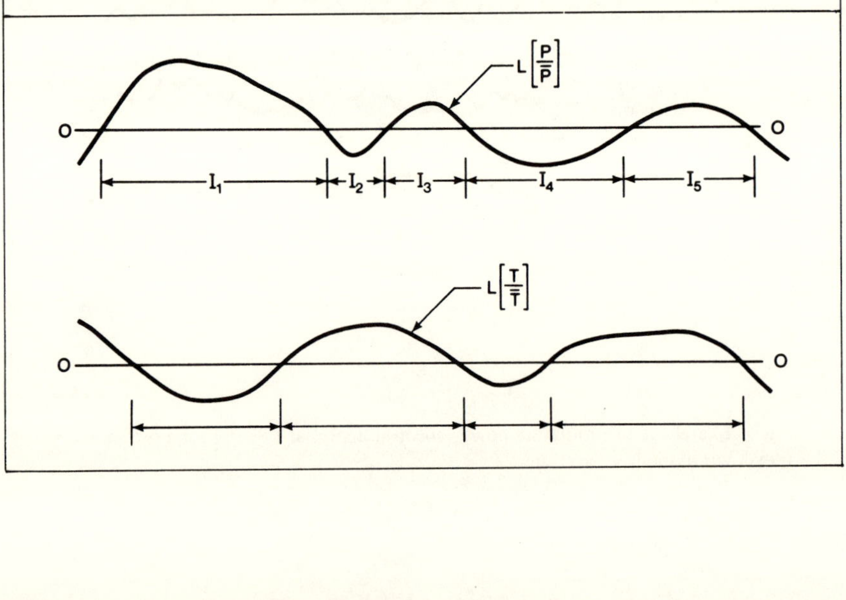
$L\left[\frac{P}{\bar{P}}\right]$
O
O
I_1
I_2
I_3
I_4
I_5
$L\left[\frac{T}{\bar{T}}\right]$
O
O

4

Table I. Depression (n = 20) vesus normals (n = 22): eyes open

		8–13 Hz	13–20 Hz	20–50 Hz
R/L shifts/s	parietal	NS	↓ *	NS
	temporal	NS	↓ **	↓ **
R/L s/shift	parietal	NS	↑ *	NS
	temporal	NS	↑ *	↑ *
Intervals:				
< 0.07 s	parietal	NS	↓ *	NS
	temporal	NS	NS	↓ *
< 0.35 s	parietal	NS	NS	NS
	temporal	NS	↓ **	↓ *
> 0.60 s	parietal	NS	NS	NS
	temporal	NS	↑ *	↑ *
Total intervals	parietal	NS	↓ *	NS
	temporal	NS	↓ *	↓ *

t test: * $p < 0.05$; ** $p < 0.025$.

Results

Depression and mania compared to normals, both showed a significant reduction of right/left shifts per second in the beta range 13–20 and 20–50 Hz (table I, II). This was true in the temporal and parietal regions for the slow beta but was only found temporally for the faster activity. Depression did not differ from normals in the alpha frequencies; however, mania exhibited significantly more right/left shifts for parietal alpha than did the normals. In schizophrenia the right/left shifts were reduced temporally only in the 20–50 Hz band (table III). Mania, depression and schizophrenia were all characterized by a greater number of intervals longer than 0.60 s in the temporal region (beta range).

When comparisons were made between mania and depression (table IV), depression and schizophrenia (table V), and mania and schizophrenia (table VI) then the significant differences occurred only in the alpha frequencies: manics showed more frequent parietal shifts than schizophrenics as did depressives when compared to schizophrenics but there were no significant differences between mania and depression.

Fig. 2. Calculation of average power ratios.

Fig. 3. Calculation of instantenous power ratios.

Fig. 4. Calculation of the intervals of lateralized EEG.

Table II. Mania (n = 21) versus normals (n = 22): eyes open

		8–13 Hz	13–20 Hz	20–50 Hz
R/L shifts/s	parietal	NS	↓ **	NS
	temporal	NS	↓ *	↓ **
R/L s/shift	parietal	NS	↑ **	NS
	temporal	NS	↑ *	↑ **
Intervals				
<0.07 s	parietal	↑ *	↓ *	NS
	temporal	NS	↓ *	↓ **
<0.35 s	parietal	NS	↓ **	NS
	temporal	NS	↓ **	↓ **
>0.60 s	parietal	NS	NS	NS
	temporal	NS	↑ **	↑ **
Total intervals	parietal	NS	↓ **	NS
	temporal	NS	↓ **	↓ **

t tests: * $p < 0.05$; ** $p < 0.025$.

Table III. Schizophrenia (n = 19) versus normals (n = 22): eyes open

		8–13 Hz	13–20 Hz	20–50 Hz
R/L shifts/s	parietal	NS	NS	NS
	temporal	NS	NS	↓ **
R/L s/shift	parietal	NS	NS	NS
	temporal	NS	NS	↑ **
Intervals				
<0.07 s	parietal	NS	NS	↓ **
	temporal	NS	NS	↓ **
<0.35 s	parietal	NS	NS	↓ *
	temporal	NS	NS	↓ **
>0.60 s	parietal	NS	NS	NS
	temporal	NS	↑ *	↑ **
Total intervals	parietal	NS	NS	↓ *
	temporal	NS	NS	↓ **

t tests: * $p < 0.05$; ** $p < 0.025$.

Table IV. Mania (n = 21) versus depression (n = 20): eyes open

		8–13 Hz	13–20 Hz	20–50 Hz
R/L shifts/s	parietal	NS	NS	NS
	temporal	NS	NS	NS
R/L s/shift	parietal	NS	NS	NS
	temporal	NS	NS	NS
Intervals				
<0.07 s	parietal	NS	NS	NS
	temporal	NS	NS	NS
<0.35 s	parietal	NS	NS	NS
	temporal	NS	NS	NS
>0.60 s	parietal	NS	NS	NS
	temporal	NS	NS	NS
Total intervals	parietal	NS	NS	NS
	temporal	NS	NS	NS

Table V. Depression (n = 20) versus schizophrenia (n = 19): eyes open

		8–13 Hz	13–20 Hz	20–50 Hz
R/L shifts/s	parietal	↑ *	NS	NS
	temporal	NS	NS	NS
R/L s/shift	parietal	↓ *	NS	NS
	temporal	NS	NS	NS
Intervals				
<0.07 s		NS	NS	NS
<0.35 s	parietal	↑ *	NS	NS
	temporal	NS	NS	NS
>0.60 s	parietal	↓ *	NS	NS
	temporal	NS	NS	NS
Total intervals	parietal	↓ *	NS	NS
	temporal	NS	NS	NS

t test: * $p < 0.05$

Table VI. Mania (n = 21) versus schizophrenia (n = 19): eyes open

		8–13 Hz	13–20 Hz	20–50 Hz
R/L shifts/s	parietal	↑ *	NS	NS
	temporal	NS	NS	NS
R/L s/shift	parietal	↓ *	NS	NS
	temporal	NS	NS	NS
Intervals				
<0.07 s	parietal	↑ *	NS	NS
	temporal	NS	NS	NS
<0.35 s	parietal	↑ *	NS	NS
	temporal	NS	NS	NS
>0.60 s	parietal	↓ **	NS	NS
	temporal	NS	NS	NS
Total intervals	parietal	↑ *	NS	NS
	temporal	NS	NS	NS

t tests: * $p < 0.05$; ** $p < 0.025$.

Table VII. Mania: before lithium (n = 6) versus after lithium (n = 6) (asymptomatic)

	8–13 Hz	13–20 Hz	20–50 Hz
Eyes open			
Intervals <0.07 s temporal	↑ *	NS	NS
Intervals >0.60 s temporal	NS	↑ *	NS
Eyes closed			
Intervals <0.07 s parietal	↑ *	NS	NS
Intervals >0.60 s temporal	NS	↓ *	NS
CV (eyes open) parietal left / right	↑ *	temp.R. ↑ * (eyes closed)	variance ↑ * temp. R. (eyes closed)
Coherence			
Magnitude PR-TR EO and EC	↓ *	↓ **	NS
PL-TR		↓ *	NS
Eyes open TR-TL	NS	↓ *	NS
log R/L coherence ratio			
EO and EC	↓ **	NS	NS

t test: * $p < 0.05$; ** $p < 0.025$.

Six manics were studied before medication, when psychotic, then after lithium therapy and symptomatic recovery. In the manic state they showed significantly more frequent right/left temporal shifts (8–13 Hz) for the intervals shorter than 0.07 s (eyes open) and had more frequent parietal shifts (0.07-s intervals; eyes closed). Further, in the manic phase, the parietal coefficient of variation was bilaterally increased but in the temporal regions this was found only on the right side. Of interest, also, was the fact that the right intrahemispheric coherence (T_r–P_r) was reduced in the alpha range during the psychotic phase, as were the crossed coherences T_r–P_l and T_r–T_l (table VII).

Conclusion

These results support the hypothesis of perturbed interhemispheric organization in the psychoses. The most general finding is that the right/left energy oscillation are slowed down in psychoses when compared to normals. There is the interesting exception of mania where the parietal oscillations are, on the other hand, increased. Because in psychosis there is an excess of cerebral energy in the fast frequencies (20–50 Hz), the significant findings are found in this frequency band alone in the psychotic-control comparison. However, this then becomes a common denominator in the within-psychosis comparisons and now the significant findings emerge in the alpha frequencies. It is noteworthy that in the case of mania the differences in the parietal oscillations found when manias were compared to normals were similar to those found when manics were compared to themselves after recovery.

References

1 Flor-Henry, P.: Lateralized temporal-limbic dysfunction and psychopathology, Ann. N.Y. Acad. Sci. *280:* 777–795 (1976).

2 Flor-Henry, P.: On certain aspects of the localization of the cerebral systems regulating and determining emotion. Biol. Psychiat. *14:* 677–698 (1979).

3 Gruzelier, J.H.; Flor-Henry, P.: Hemisphere asymmetries of function in psychopathology (Elsevier, Amsterdam 1979).

4 Editorial: Psychosis and lateralisation of the brain. Lancet *ii:* 1276–1277 (1979).

5 Beaumont, J.G.; Dimond, S.J.: Brain disconnection and schizophrenia. Br. J. Psychiat. *23:* 661 (1973).

6 Dimond, S.J.; Scammell, R.E.; Pryce, I.G.; Huws, D., et al.: Callosal transfer and left-hand anomia in schizophrenia. Biol. Psychiat. *14:* 735–739 (1979).

P. Flor-Henry, MD, University of Alberta, Alberta Hospital, Edmonton, Alta. (Canada)

Adv. biol. Psychiat., vol. 6, pp. 68–71 (Karger, Basel 1981)

Asymmetrical Frontal Lobe Function during a Transient Depressive State

Don M. Tucker

Department of Psychology, University of North Dakota; Human Nutrition Research Laboratory, Science and Education Administration, US Department of Agriculture, Grand Forks, N. Dak., USA

Evidence from a variety of sources indicates that the major forms of human psychopathology are accompanied by consistent patterns of asymmetrical function of the cerebral hemispheres. While there are a variety of methodological issues which must be addressed in this research, the theoretical significance of this asymmetry must also be considered. Observing lateralized impairment of brain function traditionally leads to the interpretation of a lateralized brain lesion. Although many instances of psychopathology may be caused or complicated by organic pathology, I suggest that evidence of asymmetrical activation and function of the two hemispheres in normal emotion has important parallels to the evidence of asymmetrical brain function in psychopathology. This research with normal emotion has led to a consideration of lateralized arousal processes in the brain, mediated by specific neurotransmitter systems, that differentially regulate the contributions of the two hemispheres to ongoing cognition. The operation of these arousal processes may be closely associated with the subjective experience of emotion [1].

Research by *Flor-Henry* [2, 3] has indicated that in contrast to a left hemisphere dysfunction in schizophrenia, patients with affective disorders show impaired right hemisphere contribution to neuropsychological task performance. Congruent findings with affective disorder patients by *Yozawitz* et al. [4] and *Bruder and Yozawitz* [5] showed a pattern of dichotic listening performance in these patients which was similar to that shown by patients with known right hemisphere lesions. Other research has shown that a right hemisphere deficit characterizes patients who are diagnosed specifically as depressed.

Examining the specific symptom of depression in this research is important given findings that when the depression is improved the right hemisphere's performance capacity may normalize. *Kronfol* et al. [6] showed that when ECT clears the depression, right hemisphere performance improves. A similar cognitive improvement specific to the right hemisphere was found following tricyclic treatment in depressed children [7]. These observations suggest a close correspondence between an individual's mood level and the right hemisphere's performance ability.

In initial research on normal emotion with college students, *Tucker* et al. [8] found that those students who reported greater depression on an adjective checklist also reported less vivid visual imagery. Questioning whether this finding may indicate a normal analogue to right hemisphere dysfunction in psychiatric depression, we attempted to manipulate mood level experimentally, then to examine measures of relative hemispheric activation and performance. We worked closely with undergraduate students to insure that the hypnotic mood induction procedures would be effective and would be an educational experience for the students. After an induction period, direct suggestions of mood level were given, taken from diagnostic descriptions of mania or depression. During the mood condition, the subjects performed an auditory attentional bias task, in which tones were presented to both ears simultaneously and the subject was asked to report which tone sounded louder. The subject also performed two cognitive tasks, one involving mental arithmetic and the other visual imagery, in counterbalanced order. The subject was then removed from the hypnotic trance, debriefed to insure the mood had cleared, then the opposite mood condition was initiated, with a parallel set of attentional and cognitive tasks.

The mood induction procedures in this research, particularly for depression, were effective, and often several minutes were required for the mood to clear. The results for the auditory attentional bias task showed symmetrical judgments of tone loudness during the euphoric mood, but a bias toward reporting the right ear as louder during the depressed mood condition. This result suggests relatively greater left than right hemisphere activation during the depressive state, and may parallel findings of asymmetrical dichotic listening performance in affective disorders [4, 5]. The results for the cognitive tasks indicated that arithmetic performance was stable across mood conditions, but imagery was impaired in depression.

It is not possible to draw clear inferences as to hemispheric performance from these simple tasks. Imagery and arithmetic differ on many features other than the requirement for lateralized processing. However, this study does indicate that the relationship between depression and poor imagery that we observed in our earlier research could be found with a transient affective state. Also, the auditory attentional bias data provide some independent indication of a relative shift in hemispheric activation during the depressive mood. To gather electrophysiological data on hemispheric activation during induced mood states we repeated our mood induction procedures with a new group of students, this time recording EEG signals from the left and right frontal (F3, F4), central (C3, C4), parietal (P3, P4), and occipital (0,1, 02) electrode sites. The EEG was amplified with low-noise, optially coupled, battery-powered amplifiers with a 0.1 time constant, and digitized at 500 samples per second. Epochs of 2 s of EEG data were Fourier analyzed; with a 2-s inter-epoch interval, power spectra for 15 epochs were generated for each 1-min recording period, the length of each of the arithmetic and imagery tasks in each mood condition. Power in the alpha band (7.5–12.5 Hz) was extracted from each power spectrum, and the mean left minus right alpha power values for each region were subjected to a mood by task repeated measures analysis of variance. The task factor was significant for the occipital region ($F = 7.49$, $p < 0.02$), in the direction consistent with previous research. The mood factor was significant only for the frontal lobes ($F = 8.34$, $p < 0.01$), with the direction of the asymmetry indicating relatively less alpha over the right frontal region during depression.

Under the assumption that alpha desynchrony indicates cortical activation, these results indicate that the depressed mood in this research was characterized by activation of the right frontal region. A similar pattern of asymmetrical frontal alpha as a function of normal emotion has been reported recently by *Davidson* [9]. Independently of our research, he found that normal subjects' reports of negative emotion in two experimental conditions were associated with activation of the right frontal region, while positive emotion appeared to be associated with greater left frontal activation.

Davidson [9] interprets the data as congruent with his view that the left hemisphere handles positive emotion, while the right hemisphere is more involved in negative emotion. This interpretation is in agreement with interpretations of the emotional effects of unilateral brain lesions recently offered by *Sackeim* et al. [10], although other interpretations of this literature are possible [1]. Since my colleagues and I observed frontal lobe activity during the same mood conditions which seemed to produce impairment of the right hemisphere's performance, we have considered whether the right frontal lobe activity may represent an inhibitory process, rather than indicating a general involvement of the right hemisphere in negative emotion.

More research and theoretical work is required to reach a definite understanding of the role of the frontal lobes in emotion. What does seem clear at this point is that particular emotions may involve asymmetrical frontal activity. That the findings of frontal asymmetry in normal emotions may be relevant to brain function in psychopathology is supported by recent EEG findings in relation to specific symptoms in depressed psychiatric patients by *Perris and Monakhov* [11] and *Perris* et al. [12]. Beta activity of the right precentral area seemed to be relevant to depressive mood, while symptoms of ruminative ideation and anxiety appeared to covary more closely with activity of the precentral region of the left hemisphere. Through further research examining the relationship of lateralized cortical activation to specific psychiatric symptoms and to chronic or transient states of emotional arousal, it may be possible to better understand those processes in the brain which support the relationship between emotional integrity and cognitive competence.

Summary

An association between a depressed mood and impaired visual imagery in normal students, observed both cross-sectionally and with experimental mood induction, may parallel the poor right hemisphere performance of psychiatric depressives. Asymmetrical frontal lobe activation found during a transient depressed mood in normals suggests that altered lateralized arousal processes in psychiatric disorders may represent pathological forms of normal emotional processes.

References

1 Tucker, D.M.: Lateral brain function, emotion and conceptualization. Psychol. Bull. *81:* 19–46 (1981).
2 Flor-Henry, P.: Lateralized temporal-limbic dysfunction and psychopathology. Ann. N.Y. Acad. Sci. *280:* 777–797 (1976).
3 Flor-Henry, P.: Psychosis, neurosis, and epilepsy: developmental and gender-related effects and their aetiological contribution. Br. J. Psychiat. *124:* 144–150 (1974).
4 Yozawitz, A.; Bruder, G.; Sutton, S.; Sharpe, L.; Gurland, B.; Fleiss, J.; Costa, L.: Dichotic perception: evidence for right hemisphere dysfunction in affective psychosis. Br. J. Psychiat. *135:* 229–237 (1979).
5 Bruder, G.E.; Yozawitz, A.: Central auditory processing and laterality in psychiatric patients; in Gruzelier, Flor-Henry, Hemisphere asymmetries of function and psychopathology (Elsevier, Amsterdam 1979).
6 Kronfol, Z.; Hamsher, K. deS.; Digre, K.; Waziri, R.: Depression and hemispheric functions: changes associated with unilateral ECT. Br. J. Psychiat. *132:* 560–567 (1978).
7 Brumback, R.A.; Staton, R.D.; Wilson, H.: Neuropsychological study of children during and after remission of endogenous depressive episodes. Percept. Mot. Skills *50:* 1163–1167 (1980).
8 Tucker, D.M.; Stenslie, C.E.; Roth, R.S.; Shearer, S.L.: Right frontal lobe activation and right hemisphere performance decrement during a depressed mood. Archs gen. Psychiat. *38:* 169–174 (1981).
9 Davidson, R.J.: Hemispheric specialization for affective processes in normals: behavioral and electrophysiological studies. Paper presented to the Society for Biological Psychiatry, 1978.
10 Sackeim, H.A.; Weiman, A.L.; Gur, R.C.; Greenberg, M.S.; Hungerbuhler, J.P.: Functional brain asymmetry in the experience of positive and negative emotions: lateralization of insult in cases of uncontrollable emotional outbursts (in preparation, 1980).
11 Perris, C.; Monakhov, K.: Depressive symptomatology and systematic structural analysis of the EEG; in Gruzelier, Flor-Henry, Hemisphere asymmetries of function and psychopathology (Elsevier, Amsterdam 1979).
12 Perris, C.; Monakhov, K.; Knorring, L. von; Botskarev, V.; Nikiforov, A.: Systematic structural analysis of the electroencephalogram of depressed patients: general principles and preliminary results of an international collaborative study. Neuropsychobiology *4:* 207–228 (1978).

Dr. D.M. Tucker, Department of Psychology, University of North Dakota,
Grand Forks, ND 58202 (USA)

Adv. biol. Psychiat., vol. 6, pp. 72–75 (Karger, Basel 1981)

Hemispheric Lateralization of Fast EEG Activity in Schizophrenia and Endogenous Depression

Jan Volavka[a], *Richard Abrams*[b], *Michael A. Taylor*[b], *Dean Reker*[a]

[a] New York University Medical Center, Department of Psychiatry, Ward's Island, N.Y.
[b] The Chicago Medical School, Department of Psychiatry and Behavioral Sciences, Chicago, Ill., USA

Evidence from neuropsychological studies appears to indicate a predominantly right temporal dysfunction in the affective psychoses, and bilateral (or predominantly left-sided) temporal lobe dysfunction in schizophrenia [*Flor-Henry,* 1976, 1979; *Taylor* et al., 1979]. *Flor-Henry* [1976] also reported that EEGs of schizophrenics have more power over the left temporal area in the 20–30 Hz band than normals; the manic-depressive patients had more power in this band than normals over both temporal areas, but the difference was somewhat more pronounced over the right than over the left side. The ratio between power in higher EEG frequency bands over the right and left temporal area (T4/T3) was greater than 1 in depressive pateints and smaller than 1 in schizophrenics [*Flor-Henry* et al., 1979]. These patterns of fast activity were interpreted to reflect a left temporal lobe dysfunction in schizophrenia and a predominantly right temporal dysfunction in depressive psychosis, thus supporting the results of neuropsychological tests. We now report results of direct comparisons between EEGs of schizophrenics and endogenous depressives. One of the purposes of our study is to compare the lateralization of high frequency activity over the temporal lobe of these patients. On the basis of the results published by *Flor-Henry* [1979], we hypothesized that: (1) the two groups would differ in their right/left ratio of EEG power over temporal areas; (2) the difference would be most expressed in the higher EEG frequencies; (3) the schizophrenic patients would show relatively more high-frequency activity over the left side (in relation to their right side); (4) the opposite would be true for the depressed patients.

The patients were consecutive admissions to an acute psychiatric treatment unit of a Veterans Administration Hospital who gave a written informed consent to participate in the study and who satisfied our criteria for schizophrenia or endogenous depression. The criteria were published elsewhere [*Abrams and Taylor,* 1979]. At the time we studied them, all depressive patients and a majority of

Table I. Right-to-left ratio of power in temporal EEG derivations (T4/T3). The power values were obtained by spectral analyses of artifact-free resting EEG. Means and standard errors of the T4/T3 ratios are displayed for the two diagnostic groups. Separate t-tests were performed for each frequency band to examine the statistical significance of the difference between the two groups.

		Frequenzy bands, Hz						
Diagnosis	VAR	0.5–3.5	3.5–7.5	7.5–12.0	12.0–18.0	18.0–24.0	24.0–35.0	35.0–51.0
Depression	$\bar{x}$	0.905	0.907	0.896	0.994	0.938	0.920	0.972
(n = 40)	SEM	0.043	0.049	0.054	0.059	0.063	0.055	0.053
Schizophrenia	$\bar{x}$	0.967	0.970	1.001	0.989	1.042	1.136	1.257
(n = 37)	SEM	0.043	0.048	0.067	0.063	0.063	0.085	0.090
	p	n.s.	n.s.	n.s.	n.s.	n.s.	$p<0.05$	$p<0.01$

schizophrenics were drug-free. There was no history of ECT in the preceding 6 months. We have so far recorded EEGs from 40 depressives (37 males, 3 females, average age 47.3) and 37 schizophrenics (32 males, 5 females, average age 43.9). Hemispheric dominance was established by several methods; the two diagnostic groups showed no significant differences on this variable. Details will be reported elsewhere.

A 5-min segment of resting EEG with eyes closed was recorded on paper and on magnetic tape. The EEG derivations which we will discuss here were left and right temporal, each referenced against linked ears (T3-A12, T4-A12). The EEGs were subjected to power spectral analyses. Artifacts were deleted by experienced encephalographers who were not aware of the patients' diagnoses. (One of the more frequent reasons for rejection of EEG segments was the presence of muscle artifacts.) These procedures resulted in two sets of data: edited and unedited results of power spectral analyses. The results of the edited (i.e. artifact-free) set are presented in table I. The power in customary frequency bands is expressed as the right/left ratio (T4/T3).

The results indicate that the schizophrenics have significantly higher T4/T3 ratio than the depressives for the frequencies 24–51 Hz. Thus, the schizophrenics have relatively more power over the right than the left temporal area at higher EEG frequencies, and they differ significantly in this respect from the depressed patients who have *less* power over the right than over the left side (the ratio is smaller than 1).

These reports support our hypotheses 1 and 2 (we did find significant differences between the temporal EEGs of the two groups, and these differences were limited to the frequencies above 24 Hz). The hypotheses 3 and 4 stand rejected; the results showed exactly the opposite of what was expected.

There are several possible explanations for the discrepancy between our results and those of *Flor-Henry* [1976, 1979]. We have deleted all muscle artifacts from the EEG; he did not and assumed that the spatial distribution of myogenic potentials over the scalp is random and therefore independent of the diagnosis. This assumption may not be correct. When we summarized the results of our *unedited* data (i.e. muscle artifacts left in), the direction of the difference between the schizophrenics and the depressives was opposite to what we observe in the edited data: the T4/T3 ratio at 24–51 Hz was *higher* in the depressed than in the schizophrenic patients [*Volavka* et al., 1979]. Thus, when we followed the procedure of *Flor-Henry* [1979] (i.e. not editing for muscle artifacts), we were able to replicate his results. It is therefore possible that the myogenic potentials over the temporal areas are not randomly lateralized. The depressed patients may have more muscle potentials over the right side, which would yield a spuriously high T4/T3 ratio at high frequencies. The lateralization of muscle activity in schizophrenia may be opposite, yielding a spuriously low T4/T3 ratio. We have no direct evidence to support these hypotheses, but such data should not be difficult to acquire. It should be noted that facial muscles show a consistent asymmetry in their action when they express emotion [*Sackeim* et al., 1978].

Another hypothesis related to the editing procedure can be postulated: there is a close time link between the occurrence of muscle potentials and the genuine EEG fast activity. These two phenomena reflect the same state (anxiety, tension). Our recording and analytical techniques cannot discriminate between the two phenomena, and by rejecting segments containing muscle potentials we may be throwing out the baby with the bath water.

Flor-Henry's [1979] patient samples were selected differently from ours: we have very few female patients due to our location at a Veterans Administration facility. This and other differences in patient selection may have contributed to the disparity of the results.

Our data imply differences between schizophrenia and endogenous depression in the lateralization of hemispheric functions. We suggest that future studies of this problem ahould employ concurrent and bilateral EEG and EMG recording from the scalp, the facial muscles, and other muscles of the head.

Summary

A group of patients with endogenous depression (N-40) was compared with a group of schizophrenics (N-37) of similar age and sex distribution. Power spectral analyses of the resting EEG from the temporal derivations were performed. The results were expressed as right/left ratios. The schizophrenics had a significantly higher right/left ratio for activity at 24 Hz and above than the depressed patients.

References

Abrams, R.; Taylor, M.A.: Differential EEG patterns in affective disorder and schizophrenia. Archs gen. Psychiat. *36:* 1355–1358 (1979).

Flor-Henry, P.: Lateralized temporal-limbic dysfunction and psychopathology. Ann. N.Y. Acad. Sci. *280:* 777–797 (1976).

Flor-Henry, P.: On certain aspects of the cerebral systems regulating and determining emotion. Biol. Psychiat. *14:* 677–698 (1979).

Flor-Henry, P.; Koles, Z.J.; Howarth, B.G.; Burton, B.: Neurophysiological studies on schizophrenia, mania, and depression; in Gruzelier, Flor-Henry, Hemisphere asymmetrics of function in psychopathology, pp. 189–222 (Elsevier, Amsterdam 1979).

Sackeim, H.A.; Gur, R.C.; Saucy, M.C.: Emotions are expressed more intensely on the left side of the face. Science *202:* 434–436 (1978).

Taylor, M.A.; Greenspan, B.; Abrams, R.: Lateralized neuropsychological dysfunction in affective disorder and schizophrenia. Am. J. Psychiat. *136:* 1031–1034 (1979).

Volavka, J.; Abrams, R.; Taylor, M.A.: EEG lateralization in schizophrenia and depression. Proc. 12th Annu. Winter Conf. on Brain Research, Elkhorn 1979.

Jan Volavka, MD, PhD, New York University at Manhattan Psychiatric Center, Ward's Island, NY 10035 (USA)

Adv. biol. Psychiat., vol. 6, pp. 76–80 (Karger, Basel 1981)

Measurement of the Inter-Hemispheral Differences as a Diagnostic Tool in Psychiatry

Milos Matousek, Carlo Capone, Masako Okawa

Department of Clinical Neurophysiology, Sahlgren Hospital,
Gothenburg, Sweden

Introduction

Among the EEG indicators which are closely related to the psychic symptoms, the inter-hemispheric relationships are of particular interest. However, the methods employed as well as the interpretation of the results vary so much [*Perris and von Knorring,* 1980] that it is rather difficult to evaluate the results so far presented. The aim of this study was to determine which clinical symptoms are most closely related to the inter-hemispheric asymmetry, and which EEG indicators are most informative. Further, the influence of medication is discussed. Certain normative data based on a healthy population of different ages are also presented in this report.

Material and Methods

The material consists of 63 EEGs from 27 patients (aged 22–45 years) with endogenous depression, 34 EEGs from 16 patients (aged 25–55 years) with subacute paranoid schizophrenia, and 373 EEGs from healthy subjects aged 11–75 years. Only individuals without any sign of organic brain pathology were included. The psychiatric symptoms were registered quantitatively using the Comprehensive Psychiatric Rating Scale (CPRS) suggested by *Åsberg* et al. [1978].

The EEGs were recorded with the subjects lying down with their eyes closed. The individuals displaying abnormalities except slight increase of diffuse theta activity were excluded. Altogether 60 s of artefact-free EEG were analyzed and the spectra belonging to eight derivations (F7-T3, F8-T4, C3-C0, C4-C0, T3-T5, T4-T6, P3-01 and P4-02) were calculated. The spectral values were converted to mean amplitudes (i.e. square root of the power) in six frequency bands (delta, theta, alpha 1, alpha 2, beta 1 and beta 2, with limits 1.5, 3.5, 7.5, 9.5, 12.5, 17.5 and 25 Hz).

Results

Magnitude of the Left/Right Ratio in Different Groups

The means and standard deviations of the left/right ratios are shown in table I, separately for individual groups. In normals, the amplitudes are lower on the left side in temporal and parieto-occipital derivations (left/right ratio <1). The relationship tends to be reversed in the anterior derivations. The ratio is almost independent of age. No significant differences between left- and right-handed individuals were found.

In the schizophrenic group, the inter-hemispheric relationships show similar gradients to those in normal subjects, but the asymmetry tends to be more pronounced. The opposite trend was found in the depressive group, where many ratios are higher than one, indicating higher amplitudes on the left side.

Correlation between the Left/Right Ratios and the Psychiatric Scores

In untreated patients with endogenous depression, a significant correlation with two or more EEG symmetry indicators was found for the following CPRS items: anxiety, apparent sadness, depression, pessimistic thoughts, muscular tension and reduced speech. Similarly, the following items correlated significantly with two or more EEG measures in the patients with schizophrenia: anxiety, hypochondric ideas, apparent sadness and depression.

When discriminant analysis was employed to separate the two patient groups, 38 out of 43 patients (88%) could be correctly classified. The left/right ratio for theta, alpha1, alpha 2 and beta 1 band in temporal and parieto-occipital derivations served as input data.

Changes of the Left/Right Ratio during Treatment

To study the influence of the drugs, the EEGs recorded during treatment with zimelidine 150–300 mg, respectively with thioridazine 100–500 mg daily were added to the material. The findings can be exemplified by the correlation between the anxiety score and the left/right ratio in the theta band. A correlation coefficient of 0.42 was obtained in temporal and –0.42 in parieto-occipital derivations for untreated patients with depression (n = 27). When the EEGs recorded during treatment were added, the corresponding values were 0.52 and –0.37 (n = 63). The partial correlation compensating for the serum concentration of zimelidine was somewhat lower but still significant (0.46 and –0.35). Similar results were obtained for other clinical items in the depression group, and also in the schizophrenic group treated with thioridazine.

The discriminant analysis applied to the whole material gave less favourable results, as compared to untreated patients. Using the same EEG variables, only 69 out of 97 patients (71%) could be correctly classified.

Table I. Left/right ratios in healthy subjects and in patients with endogenous depression and schizophrenia

	Delta	Theta	Alpha 1	Alpha 2	Beta 1	Beta 2
Normals 11–22 years (n = 317)						
Fronto-temporal	1.07 (0.30)	1.09 (0.32)	1.06 (0.48)	1.07 (0.52)	1.10 (0.61)	1.13 (0.81)
Temporal	0.92 (0.26)	0.95 (0.25)	0.87 (0.27)	0.90 (0.38)	0.94 (0.29)	1.02 (0.35)
Parieto-occipital	0.96 (0.22)	0.98 (0.17)	0.96 (0.20)	0.99 (0.27)	0.96 (0.19)	0.99 (0.25)
Normals 25–50 years (n = 26)						
Fronto-temporal	0.96 (0.12)	1.03 (0.10)	0.99 (0.18)	0.98 (0.19)	1.01 (0.17)	0.99 (0.19)
Central	1.00 (0.11)	1.00 (0.08)	0.99 (0.15)	1.01 (0.16)	1.03 (0.15)	1.03 (0.12)
Temporal	0.92 (0.15)	0.95 (0.19)	0.94 (0.27)	0.92 (0.21)	0.97 (0.23)	0.93 (0.19)
Parieto-occipital	0.92 (0.10)	0.94 (0.12)	0.94 (0.20)	0.95 (0.20)	0.93 (0.12)	0.91 (0.15)
Normals 70–75 years (n = 30)						
Fronto-temporal	0.99 (0.16)	1.05 (0.20)	0.99 (0.22)	0.98 (0.20)	0.97 (0.30)	0.98 (0.42)
Central	1.03 (0.16)	1.05 (0.16)	1.09 (0.27)	1.04 (0.22)	1.02 (0.18)	1.02 (0.16)
Temporal	0.95 (0.16)	1.00 (0.28)	0.98 (0.27)	0.97 (0.23)	0.99 (0.29)	1.05 (0.40)
Parieto-occipital	0.97 (0.21)	0.99 (0.16)	0.98 (0.30)	0.93 (0.18)	0.97 (0.15)	0.97 (0.17)
Patients with endogenous depression (n = 63)						
Fronto-temporal	1.01 (0.17)	1.05 (0.14)	1.03 (0.18)	1.03 (0.22)	1.15 (0.34)	1.16 (0.46)
Central	1.03 (0.14)	1.01 (0.10)	1.03 (0.10)	0.99 (0.15)	0.99 (0.13)	1.02 (0.14)
Temporal	0.97 (0.17)	0.98 (0.17)	1.01 (0.24)	0.98 (0.25)	1.08 (0.28)	1.22 (0.58)*
Parieto-occipital	1.04 (0.28)*	1.05 (0.18)**	1.00 (0.18)	0.99 (0.20)	1.02 (0.16)*	1.02 (0.17)**
Patients with schizophrenia (n = 34)						
Fronto-temporal	0.96 (0.13)	1.00 (0.13)	1.03 (0.12)	0.93 (0.13)	0.99 (0.19)	0.91 (0.22)
Central	1.03 (0.08)	1.03 (0.11)	1.04 (0.15)	0.93 (0.10)*	0.97 (0.08)	0.97 (0.09)*
Temporal	0.92 (0.16)	0.99 (0.18)	1.00 (0.22)	0.90 (0.16)	0.91 (0.15)	0.91 (0.16)
Parieto-occipital	0.98 (0.13)	0.98 (0.11)	0.96 (0.13)	0.89 (0.13)	0.97 (0.09)	0.95 (0.11)

In the patient group, the significant differences as compared with controls aged 25–50 years are indicated (* $p < 0.05$, ** $p < 0.01$).

Discussion

As shown in this study, the EEG ratio may increase or decrease in connection with the same change of psychopathology, depending on the EEG derivation employed. The results agree with observations reported by *Flor-Henry and Koles* [1980] who found a reversed symmetry pattern in the temporal as compared with the parietal derivations. It is interesting to note that a similar reversed pattern was observed in studies of the cerebral blood flow in the temporal and posterior areas [*Prohovnik* et al., 1980]. The topographical aspects should be borne in mind reviewing the literature. Thus, *d'Elia and Perris* [1973] as well as *Goldstein* [1975] described an increase of EEG amplitudes on the right side in depression. They used centro-parietal derivations and the laterality would probably be the opposite in temporal derivations.

The theoretical background to the relationships between the EEG laterality and psychopathology in unclear. The dominance of the hemispheres is heterogeneous, and handedness is a factor of quantitative rather than qualitative importance [*Thomas and Campos,* 1978]. The hemispheric dominance varies in connection with different tasks [*Moore,* 1980]. According to own observations [*Matousek* et al., 1980], the vigilance fluctuation can be a common denominator for the EEG symmetry and psychopathology.

Summary

The ratio between EEG amplitudes on the left and on the right side is related to the intensity of depression and anxiety. The EEG indicators show a reversed topographic pattern in depression and in schizophrenia. The contrast between the values for depression and schizophrenia suggests that the EEG symmetry measures may be of value for differential diagnosis. Unlike the conventional EEG measures, such as the amount of slow activity, the left/right ratio informs on the psychic state during treatment, being relatively independent on the serum concentration of the psychotropic drug.

References

Åsberg, M.; Perris, C.; Schalling, D.; Sedvall, G.: The CPRS – development and applications of a psychiatric rating scale. Acta psychiat. scand., suppl. 271 (1978).

d'Elia, G.; Perris, C.: Cerebral functional dominance and depression. Acta psychiat. scand. *49:* 191–197 (1973).

Flor-Henry, P.; Koles, Z.J.: EEG studies in depression, mania and normals: evidence for partial shifts of laterality in the affective psychoses. Adv. Biol. Psychiat., vol. 4, pp. 21–43 (Karger, Basel 1980).

Goldstein, L.: Time domain analysis of the EEG; in Dolce, Kunkel, CEAN computerized EEG analysis (Fisher, Stuttgart 1975).

Matousek, M.; Nyström, C.; Hallström, T.: Objectification of the antidepressive drug effect by means of less conventional EEG measures; in Radouci-Thomas, Garcin, Abstr. 12th CINP Congr. Progress in Neuro-Psychopharmacology, p. 432 (Pergamon Press, Oxford 1980).

Moore, W.H.: A study of alpha hemispheric asymmetries for verbal and nonverbal stimuli in males and females. Brain Language *9:* 338–349 (1980).

Perris, C.; L. von Knorring: Clinical neurophysiological aspects of psychopathological conditions. Adv. Biol. Psychiat., vol. 4 (Karger, Basel 1980).

Prohovnik, I.: Håkansson, K.; Risberg, J.: Observations on the functional significance of regional cerebral blood flow on 'resting' normal subjects. Neurophsychologia *18:* 203–217 (1980).

Thomas, E.G.; Campos, J.J.: The relationship of handedness to a 'lateralized' task. Neuropsychologia *16:* 511–515 (1978).

M. Matousek, MD, Department of Clinical Neurophysiology
Sahlgren Hospital, Gothenburg (Sweden)

Adv. biol. Psychiat., vol. 6, pp. 81–86 (Karger, Basel 1981)

Modifications of Sleep in Depressed Patients: Possible Physiopathological Implications

J.-M. Gaillard, G. Iorio, R. Blois, J. Richard, R. Tissot

Psychiatric Clinic of the University of Geneva (Director: Prof. *R. Tissot*), Clinique de Bel-Air, Chêne-Bourg, Switzerland

Introduction

It is now well established that sleep is modified in depressive state, not only in its total quantity, but also in its composition. Paradoxical sleep (PS) has been reported to increase or decrease. These contradictory findings are probably due to the fact that this stage was described by its total time in minutes or by its percentage with respect to total sleep. These measures can be misleading since the function of PS with respect to total sleep is not linear but parabolic [*Gaillard and Martin,* 1975]. In order to avoid this problem, we have introduced the computation of general trends of sleep stages, which are functions of total sleep time, describing the evolution of the stage under consideration during the night [*Gaillard,* 1979].

One of the most consistent modifications of the internal organization of sleep in depressed patients is the shortening of the latency of PS [*Kupfer and Forster,* 1972]. This parameter is measured by the lapse of time between sleep onset and the beginning of the first episode of PS. In primary depression, several investigators have found a value around 40 min, compared to 80–90 min in normal subjects. It should be noticed however that this latency is very rarely nil, as it is in narcolepsy. Conversely, in secondary depression, the value of this parameter is close to its value in normal subjects [*Kupfer,* 1978]. It has also been shown that the frequency of rapid eye movements in the first episode of PS is high in primary depression, contrary to normal subjects [*McPartland* et al., 1978].

A short latency of PS and a high density of rapid eye movements early in the night point to an anomaly of the distribution of this stage in depression. Therefore, we considered it worthwhile to investigate more closely its evolution as a function of sleep time. The characteristics of sleep in depressed patients have been used as hints for their classification. However, an abnormal distribution of PS not only has a semiological interest, but may give indications on the functional state of the brain mechanisms involved in the production of this stage; the same mechanisms may also be implicated in the physiopathology of depressive states.

Over the past 20 years, the catecholamine (CA) hypothesis of affective disorders has been regarded as one of the most attractive in the physiopathology of these diseases. It states that 'some, if not all, depressions are associated with an absolute or relative deficiency of catecholamines, particularly norepinephrine, at functionally important adrenergic sites in the brain' [*Schildkraut,* 1965]. In spite of a large number of investigations, very few unambiguous arguments have been proposed to support this theory and a number of reviews have recently emphasized some of the difficulties with it [*Shopsin* et al., 1974; *Mendels and Frazer,* 1974; *Luchins,* 1976; *Berger and Barchas,* 1977]. On the other hand, many experimental results, mostly in animals, have shown that brain CA systems play a role in the regulation of PS [*Jouvet,* 1972]. It is therefore reasonable to consider that anomalies in the production of this stage in depressed patients may be linked to some abnormal function of their brain CA systems.

In the rat and in man, a low dose of chlorpromazine (CPZ) enhances the production of PS, whereas a higher dose decreases it in a dose-related manner [*Kafi and Gaillard,* 1978; *Gaillard and Kafi,* 1979a, b]. The enhancement of PS after a low dose of CPZ is suppressed in the rat by pretreatment with a small dose a α-methyl-paratyrosine, and in man by a small dose of clonidine, ineffective by itself. These and other results indicate that pre- and postsynaptic receptors are involved in the regulation of PS. The aim of the present investigation was to describe the temporal organization of PS in severely depressed patients and to test the effect of CPZ.

Methods

The patients participating in this study were divided in a first group of 4 females and 2 males (22–45 years old) and a second group of 7 elderly females (66–75 years). They were of the unipolar type, and selected on the basis of a major depressive episode as defined by the research diagnostic criteria [*Spitzer* et al., 1975]. These depressive episodes were of a primary type, that is occurred in patients free of any other previous psychiatric disorder. The control group consisted in 13 normal subjects (29–72 years). Since there was no difference in the characteristics and evolution of PS in young and elderly control subjects, they were treated as a single group.

In patients all psychotropic drugs were withdrawn at least 15 days before the beginning of the experiments. The results were not significantly different between the patients receiving antidepressant drugs before and those who did not. We can thus reasonably assume that the results are not contaminated by any rebound effect which could have lasted more than 15 days. In any case, this delay of 15 days, to which the nights spent in the laboratory must be added, is the maximum tolerable without treatment for this kind of patients.

After one habituation night, the patients were recorded using standard procedures in the laboratory for 3 consecutive baseline nights under placebo, and 1 night under 0.5 mg/kg of chlorpromazine, given per os 20 min before the start of the recording. Control subjects were recorded for 2–3 nights without treatment, in the same conditions. All recordings were made on magnetic tape and processes by an automatic sleep scoring system [*Gaillard and Tissot,* 1973]. The general trends of PS were calculated as recently described [*Gaillard,* 1979].

Results

Depressed patients had a much shorter total sleep (428 vs 485 min, $p < 0.05\%$) and more awakenings during the night (11.1 vs 5.0, $p < 0.005$) than normal subjects. There was no indication of a particular predominance of this excess of waking in a given part of the night, in good agreement with the results of *Hinton* [1963]. Indices of stability of sleep, such as the number of stage shifts, were similar to the values of the control group. This, along with a normal amount of slow wave sleep (stages 3 and 4), indicates that insomnia in these depressed patients does not conform to the pattern seen in chronic primary insomnia without depressive trends, as recently described [*Gaillard,* 1978]. This insomnia is more likely due to an increased pressure of wakefulness, rather than to an instability of sleep.

The latency of PS in our group of depressed patients was 45 min; that is much shorter than the corresponding value in normals, 89 min ($p < 0.001$), and very close to the value of 39 min observed by *Kupfer* et al. [1978] in a group of 47 patients with primary depression. This short latency is an expression of a high pressure of PS at the beginning of the night. In depression, the function describing the cumulation of PS with respect to sleep time, the general trend of PS, was parallel to the normal curve and had the same positive parabolic shape, but was shifted to the left. Thus, at every moment of the night, depressed patients had on the average an excess of about 15 min of PS over normal subjects. PS appeared earlier with respect to sleep onset, but was thereafter produced at a rate similar to the control group. This particular feature could be understood as a phase advance of PS with respect to total sleep. The young and elderly groups were remarkably similar, which indicates that age is not a relevant factor in this respect.

In all our patients but one, CPZ at the dose of 0.5 mg/kg enhanced the production of PS. This enhancement was approximately the same as previously seen in normal subjects [*Gaillard and Kafi,* 1979a, b]. 1 patient of the elderly group, however, reacted quite differently: CPZ decreased markedly the production of PS. It is interesting to point out that this patient had a particularly high production of PS in baseline nights, had a severe clinical symptomatology, and was the only one clinically diagnosed as stuporous melancholia.

Discussion

It is now well accepted that a short latency of PS is very frequent in primary depression and can be considered as a biological marker in this condition [*Kupfer* et al., 1978]. We show here that this early appearance of PS in the night is followed by a production rate which is on the average similar to that of control subjects.

Many experimental results obtained in animals and in man point to a role of brain CA neurons in the executive mechanisms of PS [*Jouvet,* 1972]. Although the exact relationship of their activity to PS is still subject to controversies, several results suggest a positive correlation between them [*Gaillard and Kafi,* 1979a, b]. In other words, an enhancement of the activity of these neurons, and probably mainly of the noradrenergic neurons, results in an increase of the production of PS and vice versa. In this line of interpretation, the enhancement of the production of PS observed in depressed patients is hardly compatible with a brain CA deficiency.

However, if CA are necessary for the maintenance of PS, their role at the onset of this stage is less clear. What appears in depressives as a phase advance of PS with respect to total sleep could also result from the disturbance of a non-CA system at work during the first episode of NREM sleep, before the onset of the first episode of PS. Moreover, CA systems cannot be considered in isolation, but are affected by other neuronal networks which may modulate their activity. A disturbance of another yet unidentified system could account for the abnormal phase relationship between NREM sleep and PS. Other anomalies of rhythmic activities have been described in depressed patients, such as a phase advance of the urinary excretion of MHPG, as compared to normal subjects [*Wehr* et al., 1980].

A low dose of CPZ is considered to block preferentially presynaptic alpha receptors, which results in an enhancement of the release of the transmitter. This enhanced release is compensated for by an increased synthesis. If the CA synthesis capability of the neurons is limited to some extent, the administration of CPZ will result in a lower production of PS [*Kafi and Gaillard,* 1978]. In 12 of our patients the drug produced an increase of the production of PS, approximately of the same magnitude as in normal subjects. This result suggests that their CA neurons are able to enhance the transmitter synthesis in response to a presynaptic blockade.

Taken together, the present results indicate that the abnormal distribution of PS in depressed patients may be a phase advance of this stage with respect to total sleep. This phase disturbance may be related to some abnormal function of brain CA neurons, although the role of other non-CA systems cannot be excluded. Finally, if a disturbance exists in brain CA neurons in depression, it is probably not a mere insufficiency of transmitter synthesis or availability, but it involves a more subtle dysregulation.

Summary

It has been proposed that brain catecholaminergic systems are disturbed in depressive states, and that this disturbance may consist of an insufficient transmission in noradrenergic synapses. In order to gain some information on this point, we have recorded a group of depressed patients in baseline conditions and after a small dose of chlorpromazine. The baseline recordings confirmed the findings of other laboratories, mainly a shortened latency of paradoxical sleep (PS). A low dose of chlorpromazine enhanced the production of PS in depressed patients, as it did in normal subjects. The normal response to chlorpromazine may indicate that if a disturbance of catecholaminergic systems exists in depression, it is not merely an insufficiency of the transmitter in the synapse due to limited synthesis capabilities in the catecholaminergic neurons, but it may involve a more subtle dysregulation.

References

Berger, P.A.; Barchas, J.D.: Biochemical hypotheses of affective disorders; in Barchas, Berger, Ciaranello, Elliott, Psychopharmacology: from theory to practice, pp. 151–173 (Oxford University Press, New York 1977).

Gaillard, J.;M.: Chronic primary insomnia: possible physiopathological involvement of slow wave deficiency. Sleep *1:* 133–147 (1978).

Gaillard, J.-M.: Temporal organization of human sleep: general trends of sleep stages and their ultradian cyclic components. Encéphale *V:* 71–93 (1979).

Gaillard, J.-M.; Kafi S.: Involvement of pre- and postsynaptic recoptors in catecholaminergic control of paradoxical sleep in man. Eur. J. clin. Pharmacol. *15:* 83–89 (1979a).

Gaillard, J.-M.; Kafi, S.: Brain catecholaminergic control of paradoxical sleep: pharmacological studies; in Passouant, Oswald, Pharmacology of the states of alertness. Proc. Satellite Symp. of the 7th Int. Congr. Pharmacol., Montpellier 1978, pp. 85–94 (Pergamon Press, Oxford 1979b).

Gaillard, J.-M.; Martin, L.: Fitting of a parabolic trend to the general component of cumulative occurrence of REM sleep in man; in Levin, Koella, Sleep 1974. (Karger, Basel 1975).

Gaillard, J.-M.; Tissot, R.: Principles of automatic analysis of sleep records with a hybrid system. Comp. biomed. Res. *6:* 1–13 (1973).

Hinton, J.M.: Patterns of insomnia in depressive states. J. Neurol. Neurosurg. Psychiat. *26:* 184–189 (1963).

Jouvet, M.: The role of monoamines and acetylcholine-containing neurons in the regulation of the sleep-waking cycle. Ergebn. Physiol. *64:* 166–307 (1972).

Kafi, S.; Gaillard, J.-M.: Biphasic effect of chlorpromazine on rat paradoxical sleep: a study of dose-related mechanisms. Eur. J. Pharmacol. *49:* 251–257 (1978).

Kupfer, D.J.: Application of EEG sleep for the differential diagnosis and treatment of affective disorders. Pharmakopsychiatr. Neuro-Psychopharmakol. *11:* 17–26 (1978).

Kupfer, D.J.; Foster, G.: Interval between onset of sleep and rapid-eye-movement sleep as an indicator of depression. Lancet *ii:* 684–686 (1972).

Kupfer, D.J.; Foster, F.; Coble, P.; McPartland, R.J.; Ulrich, R.F.: The application of EEG sleep for the differential diagnosis of affective disorders. Am. J. Psychiat. *135:* 69–74 (1978).

Luchins, D.: Biogenic amines and affective disorders. A critical analysis. Int. Pharmacopsychiat. *11:* 135–149 (1976).

McPartland, R.J.; Kupfer, D.; Coble, P.; Spiker, D.; Matthews G.: REM Sleep in primary depression: a computerized analysis. Electroenceph. clin. Neurophysiol. *44:* 513–517 (1978).

Mendels, J.; Frazer, A.: Brain biogenic amine depletion and mood. Archs gen. Psychiat. *30:* 447–451 (1974).

Schildkraut, J.J.: The catecholamine hypothesis of affective disorders. A review of supporting evidence. Am. J. Psychiat. *122:* 203–217 (1965).

Shopsin, B.; Wilk, S.; Sathananthan, G.; Gershon, S.; Davis K.: Catecholamines and affective disorders revised: a critical assessment. J. nerv. ment. Dis. *158:* 369–383 (1974).

Spitzer, R.L.; Endicott J.; Robbins, E.: Research diagnostic criteria. Psychopharm. Bull. *3:* 22–25 (1975).

Wehr, T.A.; Muscettola, G.; Goodwin, F.K.: Urinary 3-methoxy-4-hydroxyphenylglycol. Circadian rhythm. Archs gen. Psychiat. *37:* 257–263 (1980).

J.-M. Gaillard, MD, Psychiatric Clinic of the University of Geneva
Clinique de Bel-Air, CH-1225 Chêne-Bourg (Switzerland)

Adv. biol. Psychiat., vol. 6, pp. 87–93 (Karger, Basel 1981)

Application of EEG Sleep in the Treatment of Depression

David J. Kupfer

Western Psychiatric Institute and Clinic, Department of Psychiatry, University of Pittsburgh, Pittsburgh, Pa., USA

Our current state of knowledge about affective disorders would lead us to conclude that these disorders entail a dysfunction in multiple systems and do not simply reflect alterations in mood. Among the most common clinical symptoms observed and considered by many to be critical in affective states several involve disturbances in regulatory systems such as hyper- or hyposomnia, increases or decreases in libido and sexual activity, as well as alterations in spontaneous motor activity [*Spitzer* et al., 1978]. Furthermore, it has been argued that all treatments effective for depression may impact directly on these regulatory disturbances even though it is at yet unclear as to what degree the restoration of these regulatory functions are required for normalization of work and social functioning. Since many of the core symptoms of affective disorder represent alterations in regulatory systems, investigators have frequently searched for makers of vulnerability and explored the interdependencies among aspects of biological and psychological functioning. Such an approach has yielded promising findings with regard to EEG sleep and abnormalities. Indeed the study of EEG sleep in affective states is now affording us an opportunity to examine, along with other biological variables, notions of how abberations in neurochemical and neuroendocrine pathways and circadian rhythms may be responsible for the various biological disturbances in depression.

To date, four features of EEG sleep patterns have been established as the most frequently observed abnormalities of depressed patients [*Hawkins,* 1979]. These include: sleep continuity disturbances, a marked reduction in delta sleep, shortened REM latency, and changes in phasic REM activity. We will restrict our attention to the two latter abnormalities in this report. The most frequent feature now reported for the majority of depressed patients (aside from a sleep continuity disturbance) appears to be the shortened REM latency (REM latency is the number of minutes from sleep onset until the onset of the first REM period) [*Kupfer and Foster,* 1972]. Short REM latency as a frequent feature of depressed patients has now been confirmed in over one dozen independent investigative groups. It is most commonly found in primary depression (be it unipolar or bipolar) as well as present in the majority of endogenously depressed inpatients or outpatients. The second REM sleep feature is the presence of increased REM activity in the beginning of the night. While REM sleep time is usually described as the number of minutes of REM sleep during the entire night's sleep, within this time period there can be wide individual variability with respect to the number and type of rapid eye movements. In general, we have found that for most depressed patients, especially older than 40 years of age, not only does the first REM period occur very early in the night but this REM period appears to be associated with a high level of REM activity, greater than is commonly seen in age-matched normal controls or in other groups of psychiatric patients. Several investigations using automated REM analysis [*McPartland* et al., 1978] as well as manual scoring techniques [*Vogel* et al., 1980] have reported an increase in REM frequency at the beginning of the night as compared to subsequent REM periods. Therefore, there is considerable evidence that depressed patients examined in a drug-free phase have baseline REM abnormalities which are manifested by a short REM latency and a maximally dense first REM period.

One question concerning the issue of increased REM density and REM latency are the reported age relationships. In one study within a group of 27 nonpsychotic drug-free short REM latency depressed inpatients, a young subgroup (averaging 31 years of age) was compared to an older subgroup (averaging 53 years of age). Regardless of sleep continuity differences in the subgroups, the first REM period was marked by higher REM activity when compared to the second REM period [*Kupfer* et al., submitted]. These findings demonstrated that even in patients younger than 40 years of age with short REM latency the first REM period is associated with greater amounts of REM activity. Thus, it would appear that the short REM latency and the increased REM density might be found in primary depression regardless of age.

This specific notion of a 'V shaped curve' between the first to the second to the third REM period was pursued further in an investigation of 120 primary depressed inpatients in which 84 patients met criteria for endogenous depression. Analysis of the endogenous versus nonendogenous groups revealed that despite the similar age and overall level of severity, several sleep characteristics differentiated the groups: degree of sleep continuity disturbances, shorter REM latency and a more pronounced REM density shift to the early half of the night. Despite no differences in overall REM time of individual REM periods between the two subgroups of patients (table I), REM activity and REM density (ratio of REM activity to REM time) demonstrated significant differences both across REM periods and across groups. With respect to REM activity, REM activity was significantly higher in the first REM period ($p < 0.05$) and in the third REM period ($p < 0.01$) in the endogenous group as compared to the nonendogenous group.

Table I. REM sleep patterning in primary depression

	Individual REM periods		
	1	2	3
REM time[1]			
Nonendogenous (n = 36)	17.9 ± 2.1	24.5 ± 1.9	22.1 ± 1.4
Endogenous (n = 84)	22.8 ± 1.6	19.9 ± 1.5	24.6 ± 1.4
REM activity[2]			
Nonendogenous (n = 36)	22.9 ± 3.8	28.0 ± 2.7	26.3 ± 1.9
Endogenous (n = 84)	35.1 ± 3.3	25.6 ± 2.6	35.8 ± 2.7
REM density[3]			
Nonendogenous (n = 36)	110.8 ± 11.1	112.9 ± 6.1	126.1 ± 9.3
Endogenous (n = 84)	142.1 ± 8.2	124.1 ± 7.7	144.5 ± 8.6

[1] REM time: not significant between the two groups.
[2] REM activity: $p < 0.05$ between the 1st REM periods of the two groups. $p < 0.05$ between the 3rd REM periods of the two groups.
[3] REM density (REM activity/REM time): $p < 0.05$ between the 1st REM periods of the two groups.

While there were no differences in REM activity across REM periods for the nonendogenous group, however, the endogenous group showed both a significant decrease between the first and second REM periods ($p < 0.05$) and a significant increase between the second and third REM periods ($p < 0.001$). Similar findings were present for the REM density measures. This data supported a differentiation between endogenous depressives and nonendogenous depressives with respect to the REM patterning across the night.

Significant differences in REM latency between endogenous depressed patients and nonendogenous depressed patients even when controlling for age have also been shown in 67 nonpsychotic depressed patients. Even though there is a significant relationship between REM latency and age in that the older depressed patients generally have shorter REM latencies as compared to younger depressed patients it would appear that between the ages of 26 and 50 endogenously depressed patients have a significantly shorter REM latency than nonendogenously depressed patients regardless of age.

Further investigation of biologic abnormalities in the first half of the night need the following refinements: the application of a delta sleep analyzer as well as monitoring of various neuroendocrine variables such as growth hormone, prolactin and cortisol. In order to explore possible rhythmic changes between neuroendocrine and sleep patterning in the first half of the night, studies are being conducted in individual patients with continuous all night monitoring of sleep and neuroendocrine functioning.

Whether various EEG pattern changes have predictive value or even correlative value for treatment strategies is another major objective. A considerable body of work in our laboratory has demonstrated repeatedly significant correlations between baseline REM latency in depressed patients and ultimate clinical response. The lowest and most persistently reduced REM latencies found consistently in delusional patients are generally associated with higher levels of severity and, unless treated with psychopharmacologic interventions, patients with such short REM latencies show little clinical improvement even over a 5-week period of hospitalization.

When sleep correlates of clinical response in primary depression are examined, comparison between sleep variables and clinical course during different time periods of treatment establish that the early sleep changes on amitriptyline correlate most highly with the final clinical rating at 4 weeks of treatment [*Kupfer* et al., 1980]. Comparing the sleep of the baseline period, drug nights on 50 mg and later on 150 mg, to the clinical response in 30 patients, the best predictive set (REM latency and sleep onset difficulty) for clinical response appear to be drug nights 1 and 2. A multiple regression equation generated from four sleep variables on the first drug nights highly correlated with the final clinical response. That is, patients whose immediate response to amitriptyline including lengthening of REM latency, reduction of sleep onset difficulty and 2-REM sleep and increased sleep efficiency showed the best clinical response 4 weeks later. These findings on 30 patients were confirmatory of previous data on EEG sleep measures in the early stages of antidepressant drug treatment in a pilot group of 18 patients in which a flexible dose of 150–200 mg was administered in the course of the first 2 nights demonstrating that the immediate sleep changes on the early dose demonstrated a relationship with final clinical response [*Kupfer* et al., 1976]. In 34 drug-free patients with primary endogenous depression treated with amitriptyline, the application of EEG sleep criteria alone was more significant than clinical status alone in the prediction of clinical response. Prolonged REM latency and reduced sleep onset difficulty following the administration of amitriptyline were the main sleep variables contributing to this prediction equation. This data pointed to a strong relationship between clinical outcome in patients with endogenous depression and their psychobiological profile after a 'pharmacologic probe' with a tricyclic antidepressant [*Kupfer* et al., 1981].

In order to test whether such predictions can be easily replicated, we have recently examined 46 depressed patients who were treated with amitriptyline between the ages of 31 and 65. The sleep variables, sleep onset difficulty and REM latency again demonstrated significant relationships with the final clinical response. Application of the 'jacknife' statistical technique along with the multiple regression strategy confirmed the significant multiple correlations between selective sleep variables and clinical response in the order of the 0.45–0.60 range. The addition of only one clinical variable, agitation, improved the prediction equation. Thus, it would appear that the reduction of sleep latency and prolongation of REM latency are definite early signs of clinical improvement.

Recently, studies have been completed on outpatients followed for 18 months with monthly evaluations including EEG sleep studies. Our tentative conclusions from this small sample of 10 patients are that patients maintained on tricyclic antidepressants continue to show considerable REM suppression and REM sleep alterations similar to the immediate sleep effects of tricyclic antidepressants; that the sleep changes are dose-related even during chronic tricyclic administration; and that patients withdrawn from tricyclics may demonstrate short REM latencies, suggesting that short REM latency in partially remitted patients may reflect a level of vulnerability.

While there are a number of unanswered questions regarding the use of EEG sleep measures in the prediction of treatment response among depressed patients, the significant correlation of a measure of sleep disturbance with a particular time in the course of the depressive episode might represent a powerful tool for understanding treatment course and prognosis in depression. We feel that our present findings represent an important step, be it a small one, in understanding the psychobiology of depression. Alterations in circadian rhythms in depressed patients have been suggested as explanations for various biological abnormalities associated with depression, including disturbances in sleep, motor activity, and endocrine function. It has also been proposed that sleep deprivation, which is capable of inducing transient remission of depression, slows or delays patients' circadian temperature rhythms [*Wever,* 1978]. In a similar way it has been suggested that procedures that advance the patients' environmental schedule relative to their circadian rhythms also abolish differences in timing and, therefore, improve depressed mood at least transiently [*Wehr* et al., 1979]. Clinical evidence to support such theories is derived from the data demonstrating the immediate prolongation of REM latency by amitriptyline which may represent both cholinergic actions as well as a delay in REM sleep and therefore a change in the ultradian cycling of REM sleep. Finally, the *Gillin* et al. [1978] and *Sitaram* et al. [1980] studies using cholingergic probes and the 'cholinergic REM induction test' have suggested that the action of physostigmine and arecoline on REM sleep timing (the onset of REM periods) points to a cholinergic mechanism which may be responsible for the short REM latency. This theory is furthr supported by the sensitivity of depressed patients to infusions of arecoline during depressed episodes as well as during states of remission [*Sitaram* et al., 1980], suggesting a level of vulnerability. These results would be consistent with the hypothesis that cholinergic mechanisms maintain arousal and induce REM sleep but do not control the duration of REM sleep. Against this body of evidence in support of cholinergic mechanisms is data showing that REM latency can be prolonged by non-anticholinergic tricyclic antidepressants [unpublished data] and that long-term prolongation of REM latency can be observed with continued administration of amitriptyline for periods of 6 months to 2 years despite the lack of other 'cholingergic' effects.

In summary, we have presented several sets of data which are intended to shed light on aspects of the REM sleep abnormalities in depression. It is clear that increased attention should be devoted to the interactions of age and diagnostic specificity with these sleep findings, as well as the further delineation of REM sleep patterning over the entire night. At the present time, none of the proposed theories, reciprocal oscillators, free-running and/or phase advance nor cholinergic hypotheses adequately explain the available data. Nevertheless, they represent important and innovative steps which may lead to an increased understanding of the pathophysiology of depression.

Summary

Considerable evidence exists for the presence of EEG sleep abnormalities in primary depressive disorders. Circadian or ultradian rhythm abnormalities in REM sleep, possibly related to neuroendocrine alterations, as well as generator-inhibitor oscillators involved in neurochemical pathways, especially cholinergic ones, are most frequently offered as explanations. While attention was initially devoted to sleep continuity and delta sleep alterations, the more recent focus on the REM sleep changes has emphasized the frequency of the shortened REM latency and increased REM activity (especially in the first half of the night). New EEG sleep data including automated REM analysis derived from depressed patients over an extensive age range prior to treatment, during treatment of the acute episode, and maintenance follow-up are presented in an attempt to shed further light on our understanding of the pathophysiology of sleep disturbances in affective disorders. The availability of longitudinal EEG sleep studies on depressed patients in remission represents a new direction for exploring interrelationships among vulnerability, early signs of relapse, EEG sleep abnormalities, and tricyclic drug treatment.

References

Gillin, J.C.; Mendelson, W.B.; Sitaram, N.; Wyatt, R.J.: The neuropharmacology of sleep and wakefulness. Annu. Rev. Pharmacol. Toxicol. *18:* 563–579 (1978).

Hawkins, D.R.: Sleep and depression. Psychiat.. Ann. *9:* 391–350 (1979).

Kupfer, D.J.; Coble, P.A.; Spiker, D.G.; Neil, J.F.; Shaw, D.H.: REM sleep and depression. Am. J. Psychiat. (submitted, 1980).

Kupfer, D.J.; Foster, F.G.: Interval between onset of sleep and rapid eye movement sleep as an indicator of depression. Lancet *ii:* 684–686 (1972).

Kupfer, D.J.; Foster, F.G., Reich, L.; Thompson, K.S.; Weiss, B.: EEG sleep changes as predictors in depression. Am. J. Psychiat. *133:* 622–626 (1976).

Kupfer, D.J.; Spiker, D.G.; Coble, P.A.; Neil, J.F.; Ulrich, R.; Shaw, D.H.: Depression, EEG sleep and clinical response. Compreh. Psychiat. *21:* 212–220 (1980).

Kupfer, D.J.; Spiker, D.G.; Coble, P.A.; Neil, J.F.; Ulrich, R.; Shaw, D.H.: Sleep and treatment prediction in endogenous depression. Am. J. Psychiat. *138:* 429–434 (1981).

McPartland, R.J.; Kupfer, D.J.; Coble, P.A.; Spiker, D.G.; Matthews, G.: REM sleep in primary depression: a computerized analysis. Electroenceph. clin. Neurophysiol. *44:* 513–517 (1978).

Spitzer, R.L.; Endicott, J.; Robins, E.: Research diagnostic criteria: rationality and reliability. Archs gen. Psychiat. *38:* 773–780 (1978).

Sitaram, N.; Nurnberger, J.I.; Gershon, E.S.: Faster cholinergic REM sleep induction in euthymic patients with primary affective illness. Science *208:* 200–202 (1980).

Vogel, G.W.; Vogel, F.; McAbee, R.S.; Thurmond, A.J.: Improvement of depression by REM sleep deprivation. Archs gen. Psychiat. *37:* 247–253 (1980).

Wehr, T.A.; Wirz-Justice, A.; Goodwin, F.K.; Duncan, W.; Gillin, J.C.: Phase advance of the sleep-wake cycle as an antidepressant. Science *206:* 710–713 (1979).

Wever, R.: Grundlagen der Tagesperiodik beim Menschen; in Heimann, Pflug, Rhythmus Probleme in der Psychiatrie, pp. 1–23 (Fischer, 1978).

D.J. Kupfer, MD, Western Psychiatric Institute and Clinic, Department of Psychiatry, University of Pittsburgh, 3811 O'Hara Street, Pittsburgh, PA 15261 (USA)

Adv. biol. Psychiat., vol. 6, pp. 94–101 (Karger, Basel 1981)

Changes in Motoric Variables Related to Sleeplessness in Psychotic Depressives[1]

P. Pinelli

Research Insitute for Neuropsychiatric Diseases, University of Pavia, Pavia, Italy

Different psychophysiological variables secured by corresponding serotoninergic subsystems have been shown to change during blocking of tha active reuptake of released serotonin by the presynaptic neurone [*Pinelli* et al., 1979]. *Mandell and Knapp* [1979] have observed how 'degree of attentiveness, sleepiness, temperature, pain, anger, inclination to be active, appetitional behaviors are modifiable by serotonin'. According to their interpretation the vector sum of the feelings of these phenomena could determine mood which therefore 'is nonexistent as a property per se', but 'may be an emergent property'.

Usual clinical experience indicates that increase in depressive mood can be accompanied by augmentation or reduction in motor activities. These opposite behavioral effects on one apparently identical variable ('inclination to be active') completely invalidate the hypothesis of the interdependence of the variables from their vector sum or makes one suppose that the 'single phenomena' may be substained or influenced by different biochemical subsystems or processes anyway. On the other hand, 'inclination to be active' may partially cover the concept of alertness reaction and orienting response, which are known to be enhanced by anxiety. Anxiety may often coexist with depressive mood and it can affect the reaction time and the movement time in a diphasic way [*Pinelli,* 1966].

For all these reasons we have considered the investigation of motoric functions and their correlation to the clinically evaluated resultant motor activity as a preliminary point for investigation of their correlation with other variables in somatic depressives. Among these, variable degrees of sleepiness must also be considered since it would play a primary role at least during the recovery of depression [*Vogel* et al., 1980].

[1] This research was carried out with the financial support of CNR (80–00537–04).

Method

We have investigated neurophysiological parameters related to 'inclination to be active' in 74 unipolar depressive patients.

Subjects
We investigated two groups of endogenous unipolar depressive patients during admission to the clinic because of a psychotic episode. The patients included in this research were found to be responsive to amitriptyline treatment with blood drug levels monitored [*Corona and Bonferoni,* 1976]. Some of them were also investigated during the recovery phase. The agitated-anxious depressive group consisted of 34 females and 14 males with a mean age of 41 years (range: 29–66 years, and the retarded depression group consisted of 21 females and 5 males with a mean age of 44 years (28–71). The normal controls (11) were males with an age range between 24 and 48 years.

Prior to testing, the depressed patients were left without any drug treatment for 4 days. All depressives presented with endogenous characteristics, unipolar type, according to Perris criteria. The classification into retarded (r) or agitated (a) group was carried out following the evaluation of Hamilton items, respectively 7th and 8th (for r) and 9th and 10th (for a) as it has been specified in a previous paper [*Bezzi* et al., 1981].

Physiological Recording and Data Quantification
EEG Record of Sleep. Recording of EEG during sleep and its classifications were carried out as described by *Kupfer and Foster* [1978]; two successive night records were performed for each patient. The degree of sleeplessness (– S) was quantified on a 9-point scale according to the following measurements:

I.	Total sleep time (TST)	<350 min >300 min = 1
		<300 min >250 min = 2
		<250 min = 3
II.	Awakenings after slepp onset	N = 1–2 = 1
		N = 3–4 = 2
		N > 4 = 3
III.	(Stages 3 and 4) % TST	25–15% = 1
		14–10% = 2
		<10% = 3

Serial Choice Reaction Test According to Bjerner's Methodology. Simultaneously with EEG we recorded the reactions performed by the subject just after acoustic stimuli randomly delivered by himself; the arm position was adjusted and fixed with the elbow at the same level of the switching apparatus. The technique has been described before by *Bjerner* [1949], *Pinelli* [1959] and *Bezzi* et al. [1981]. In this way one can measure reaction times, intervals between reactions, wrong reactions, delayed reactions, and of course the number of reactions during the whole time of testing (12 min according to *Bjerner's* [1949] suggestion).

Ratio between EMG Activity at Rest and EMG of the Reaction. Simple reactions to one acoustic stimulus were registered by EMG. The value of mean anplitude of the action potentials from biceps brachii and triceps brachii in the 50 ms corresponding to the response was measured (R) and divided by the mean amplitude of the action potentials in the 50 ms piece of tracing prior to the appearance of the stimulus (B). Values >10 were included in notation 10. This ratio R/B was proportional to the ability of the subject to perform specific temporal innervation of agonistic muscles. Normal people better prepared to react presented the highest values of R/B [*Bezzi* et al., 1981].

Results

Bjerner Test

The Results in normals and patients are given in table I. Normal subjects could be subdivided into 2 groups: some (8) performed the test as quick as possible (speed-concerned subjects – Sc); the others (3) were more concerned with the exactness of the performance (exactness- concerned subjects – Ec).

Agitated depressives could be divided into two groups: some (23%) did a poor performance with slow reactivity and long pauses throughout the test execution (slow-reacting patients – SR); the others performed a good deal or nearly normal reactions, interrupted by some long pauses and some Bjerner's delayed reactions (normal-reacting patients with phases of delayed reactions – NDr).

Retarded depressives showed a very poor ability to react and interrupted the performance after several minutes: some (81%) could carry out only very slow reactions (steady slow-reacting patients – SSr); several could perform a quick series of reactions but during very short periods and with many errors (slow-reacting patients with paradoxical acceleration – SPAr).

As far the significance of mean time reaction changes is concerned, the results of *Lapierre and Butter* [1980] are confirmed; also in the serial choice reaction test there was a statistically significant increase in the retarded group (+193%) but this variable (t) did not significantly differentiate the retarded group from the agitated depressives: the difference was of the order of 35% and lower than the standard deviation anyway (which greatly exceeded 50%).

The histogram of the total number of reactions in 12 min (N) is given in figure 1. In the group of agitated depressives (43 patients) a bimodal distribution was evident with a peak at 100–150 N, corresponding to the range of the retarded patients and the second peak at 350–400. The hypothetic explanation for the first peak of low N could be searched with reference to two conditions: one related to long-lasting blocking effects from continuous over-flow of central impulses which could be obviously ascribed to an innervation diffusely involving in an equal rate both agonist and antagonist muscles; the other condition could be related to the temporary lack of impulses, which could be responsible for phases of long pauses and delayed reactions. The last functional failure has been found to characterize phases of sleep and effects of sleep deprivation [*Bezzi* et al., 1981].

Table I. Bjerner test: mean values

	Normals (n = 11 ♂)		Agitated D (n = 34 ♀ + 14 ♂)		Retarded D (n = 21 ♀ + 5 ♂)	
	I Sc (8)	II Ec (3)	I Sr (11)	II NDr (37)	I SSr (21)	II SPAr (5)
Mean reaction time, s	0.63	0.67	1.3	0.95	2.1	1.2
Pauses: mean value, s	0.5	0.75	1.9	1.1	4.3	1.6
Maximum reaction time, s	1.5	0.9	3.0	4.5	8	3.4
Total number of reactions in 12 min	564	498	124	340	61 (<12 min)	128 (<12 min)
Errors, %	2–5	1–2	6	5	8	18

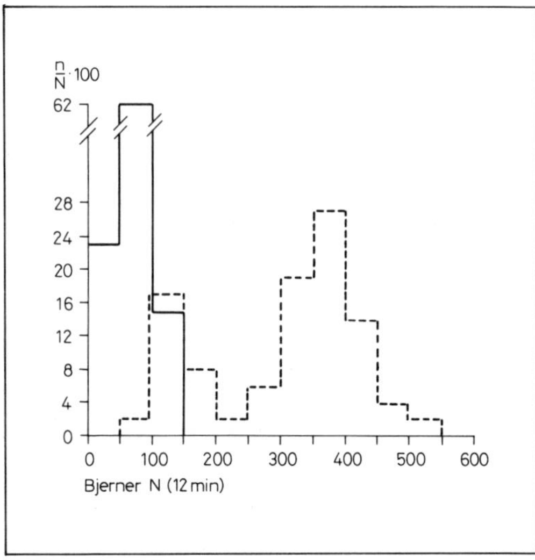

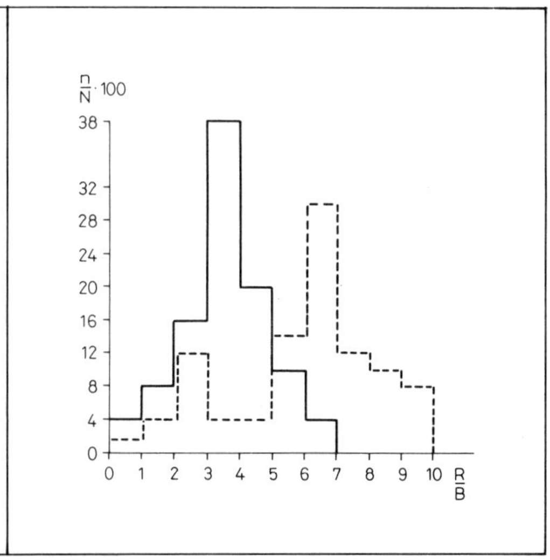

2

Fig. 1. Bjerner N in psychotic depressive patients. —— = Retarded (n = 19; r > 3.5); – – – = agitated (n = 43; a > 3.5).

Fig. 2. R/B in psychotic depressive patients. —— = Retarded (n = 26; r > 3.5); – – – = agitated (n = 48; a > 3.5).

Degree of Sleeplessness (–S) and Bjerner's Test (N)

The research was carried out in 13 depressive patients. No linear relationship was found between –S and N. Some patients in which sleep was greatly reduced showed a low N of reactions; but in some of them the N of reactions was nearly normal.

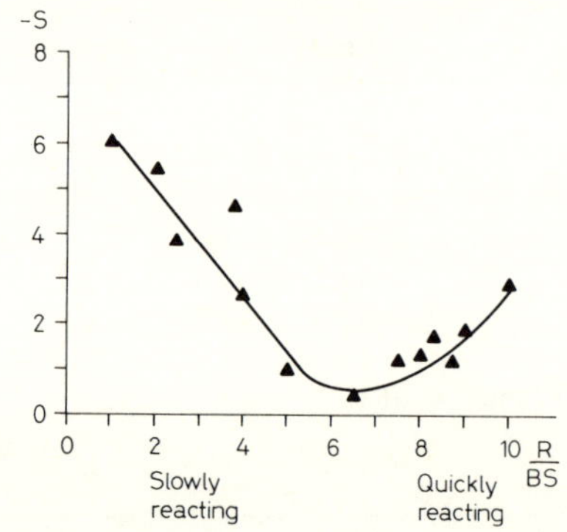

Fig. 3. Sleeplessness (−S) versus ability to get involved in movement (R/B) in psychotic depressive patients. TST: 1−3; Aw.: 1−3; % stages 3 and 4: 1−3.

Pattern of Motor Set and Reactivity

To discriminate between the two conditions of motor overinnervation or of occurrence of pauses with lack of innervation, we had to apply to EMG investigation since the Bjerner technique itself seems inadequate. The ratio R/B was chosen as one quantitative variable useful to express the state of motor innervation at rest and during the execution of reactions; of course its full meaning can be better appreciated if it is integrated with the reaction time, number of reactions, and diffusion of innervation to antagonistic muscles. Nevertheless, it yielded useful information.

The histogram of R/B values in 'retarded' and in 'agitated' depressives (fig. 2) shows that the motor basic processes are the same (i.e. high values of B in relation to R) in retarded patients and in a small number of agitated depressives (20%). In fact we found that all retarded or agitated depressives with R/B < 5 had a Bjerner N < 200. This proves that retarded patients are poorly reacting because of an overinnervation leading to a negativistic or withdrawn condition; the same was true for the 20% of agitated depressives characterized by a low number of reactions. In conclusion, among patients with the same degree of overinnervation occurring in basal conditions, some look like retarded depressives and others appear to belong to the clinical group of agitated depressives. On the other hand, a condition of delayed reaction, of the type of that shown by Bjerner following sleep deprivation, could be recognized in the group of agitated depressives with higher N of reactions.

Correlations between Sleeplessness and Neurophysiological Parameters

A correlation of parabolic-like type was found between the degree of sleeplessness and R/B (fig. 3). The highest degree of sleeplessness was found in retarded depressives and some agitated depressives with a greatly decreased number of reactions. A Bjerner type of sleep deprivation effect was found only in some patients with a high R/B ratio.

Discussion

The analysis of the Bjerner serial choice reaction test together with the electromyographical recording of the motoric set seems to offer some promising clues for a better evaluation of the psychomotor state of depressives. In previous research we have seen [*Bezzi* et al., 1981] that the ratio of electromyographical activity at rest, during the preparatory phase (basal activity B) related to the activity subserving the reaction (R), showed a negative correlation with the pain threshold which in turn is proportional to the withdrawn reflex. This result was interpreted in favor of a compensative nature of the basal activity in this type of patient: namely the abnormally lower reactivity of the acute prompt defense system to painful stimuli is compensated by a higher level of continuous withdrawn preparatory activity. The interference was drawn that the measure of these variables should give a closer definition of the functional factors contributing to the production (in a pathogenetic way) or to the shapening (in a pathoplastic way) of the psychomotor symptomatological features of the disease. In fact we have now found that retardation in depressives appears to be related to diffuse basal overinnervation, a pattern which, on the other hand, appears with identical features also in 20% of agitated depressives. This fact excludes the existence of a simple bipolar continuum between retardation and agitation. Its interpretation required not only the application of an endurance test (Bjerner serial reactions) which enabled us to analyze, besides reaction times, the ability to move from one act to the next one, but also the clinical observation of the amount of spontaneous activity (9th Hamilton's item). In fact we must consider two factors in the determination of the psychomotor state. One factor is represented by the ability to specifically and timely innervate agonistic muscles; we will call it factor R or *prompt reactivity.* The second factor corresponds to the ability to maintain a certain postural state against driving to change (i.e. against motor restlessness): we will call it factor P or *postural maintenence.* One subject can indeed lose his ability to react selectively (–factor R) while the preserved postural factor is released (+factor P); this demonstrates a state of immobility with retarded reactivity. On the other hand, one patient besides suffering from lack of Factor R can also lose the ability to maintain a posture; this demonstrates a state of agitation with retarded reactivity.

It is worthwhile recalling that the same is true even in the area of neurological motoric disorders: some patients may be affected by akinesia with block in starting of action whereas some other akinetic patients may also suffer from akathisia, a need to move the extremities, which is sometimes in fact confused with anxiety or agitation [*Windeleman,* 1961].

Factor R can be measured in function of the value of reaction time (t), ability to reach low or null activity (B) in the preparatory phase, and to move to the next reactions (N); so

$$R = \frac{1}{t(s) + B(\mu V)} + N.$$

On the other hand, factor P can be measured by the inverse ratio of the number of spontaneous purposeless movements which can be recorded by means of *Kripke's* [1978] and *Van Zerssen's* [1979] methods. Generally a high P coexists with high R (low B and high endurance), but it may also coexist with high B and low endurance. This proves the functional independence of the two factors, a dissociation which is in favor of correspondingly different systems providing their biochemical substratum. There are some trends in biological psychiatry for a prevalent mediation of serotoninergic subsystems for factor P and of dopaminergic and adrenergic subsystems for factor R; but the neuropathological research shows a much more complex situation with the intervention also of cholinergic, gabaergic and peptidergic subsystems. Anyway the individuation of the two factors P and R makes it possible to better approach the study of the relationship between motoric variables and sleep disturbances. In some agitated depressives with a relatively slight decrease in N of reactions we have recorded some long pauses and delayed reactions of the type produced by sleep deprivation. Since these patients suffered from a rather high degree of sleeplessness these periods of functional failure in the test could be explained as an effect of sleep. However, the meaning of this 'sleep deprivation' effect for the final symptomatology of depression remains of limited value since it appears only in a small percentage of patients. Moreover, we cannot neglect that the dominant feature in these patients is not represented by sleeplessness but rather by agitation anxiety.

The findings of a high degree of sleeplessness not only in retarded depressives (low R and high P) and agitated (low P) with low R but also in agitated depressives (low P) with high R offer a clearer demonstration of an independent course of the amount of sleep with respect to the other functional troubles that we have investigated in depressives: particularly a cause-effect relationship is hardly conceivable. On the contrary, psychophysiologic-dependent variables can be thought to be related to different neural subsystems, some of which are differently affected in the different types of depressions; consequently the change affecting the control of sleep oscillators [*Vogel* et al., 1980] can only be thought to represent the primary pathophysiogenetic event, but it fails to explain the large variety of effects.

References

Bezzi, G.; Pinelli, P.; Tosca, P.: Effects of sleep deprivation on motor reactivity and pain threshold in unipolar depression. Psychiatria clin. (to be published, 1981).

Bjerner, B.O.: Alpha depression and lowered pulse rate during delayed actions in a serial reaction test. A study in sleep deprivation. Acta physiol. scand. *19:* suppl. 65 (1949).

Corona, G.L.; Bonferoni, B.: Simultaneous determination of therapeutic levels of amitriptyline and nortriptyline in plasma by gas-liquid chromatography. J. Chromat. *124:* 401–404 (1976).

Kupfer, D.J.; Foster, F.G.: EEG sleep and depression; in Williams, Karacan, Sleep disorders: diagnosis and treatment, pp. 163–204 (Wiley, New York 1978).

Lapierre, Y.D.; Butter, H.J.: Agitated and retarded depression. A clinical psychophysiological evaluation. Neuropsychobiology *6:* 217–223 (1980).

Mandell, A.J.; Knapp, S.: Asymmetry and mood, emergent properties of serotonin regulation. Archs gen. Psychiat. *36:* 909–915 (1979).

Mowbray, R.M.; The Hamilton Rating Scale for depression: a factor analysis. Psychol. Med. *2:* 272–280 (1972).

Pinelli, P.: Sonno, sogno, ipnosi (Cortina, Pavia-Milano 1959).

Pinelli, P.: Interessi attuali dello studio del 'riflesso preparato' di Exner-Cattel e della reazione di rilassamento. Riv. sper. Freniat. Med. leg. Alien. ment. *88:* 426–450 (1966).

Pinelli, P.; Zerbi, F.; Fenoglio, L.; Corona, G.L.: Blood 5-hydroxytryptamine (5-HT), sleep, pain experience, depressions: time-course effects of amitriptyline treatment. Ital. J. neurol. Sci. *1:* 7–13 (1979).

Vogel, G.; Vogel, F.; McAbee-Thurmond, A.J.: Improvement of depression by REM sleep deprivation. Archs gen. Psychiat. *37:* 247–253 (1980).

Windelman, N.W. (1961); cited in Mowbray (1972).

Paolo Pinelli, MD, Istituto di Neurologia, via Palestro 3, I-27100 Pavia (Italy)

Adv. biol. Psychiat., vol. 6, pp. 102–108 (Karger, Basel 1981)

Dependence between Cerebral Metabolism and Blood Flow as Reflected in the Quantitative EEG

A Clinical Review

Ilmar A. Sulg, Kyösti A. Sotaniemi, Uolevi Tolonen, Eero Hokkanen
Departments of Neurology and Clinical Neurophysiology,
University Central Hospital, Oulu, Finland

Introduction

Ever since the EEG was detected and developed to a valuable tool for studies on brain activity, there has been accumulating evidence about a close coupling between electrical activity, blood flow and metabolic activity of the brain. With the advent of quantitative techniques in measurement of cerebral blood flow (CBF) and cerebral metabolic activity rate (CMA) it became possible to study statistical relationships between these parameters. To the most reliable method for measurement of regional CBF (rCBF) by means of intracarotide injection of isotopes [*Lassen and Ingvar,* 1961] has been later added noninvasive techniques, where isotopes are administered by inhalation or by intravenous injection. These methods have lower resolution and reliability, but measurements can be, if necessary, repeated without any harm to the patient.

QEEG, CBF and CMA from the Clinical Point of View

Since reliable methods for measurement of CBF and CMA are now available, systematic studies by means of quantitatively analyzed EEG (QEEG) have offered new information about relationships between these cerebral variables. *Obrist* et al. [1963], being the first in statistical analysis of QEEG/CBF/CMA-interdependence, were able to show that in natural aging there is no major change neither in the EEG nor in the CBF. In a matched age group of psychiatric patients, however, there was found significant slowing of the EEG parallel to decrease of CBF and CMA [*Obrist* et al., 1963]. Statistical significance of EEG dependence was higher on the CMA than on the CBF. Beginning from about 1965, *Ingvar* and his group have contributed essentially to the knowledge of the

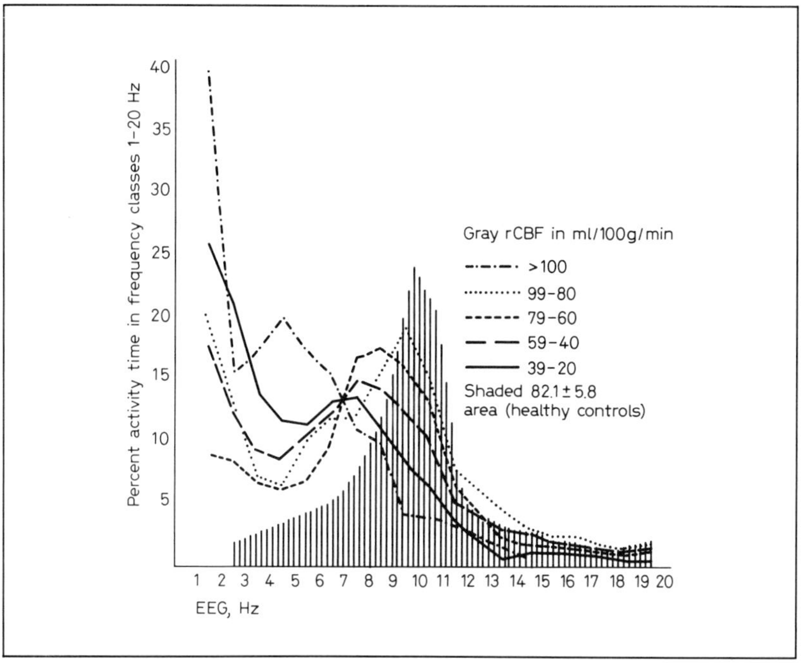

Fig. 1. Relationships between amount of EEG activity and cerebral blood flow. EEG has been recorded from parieto-occipital area and quantified by means of period analysis. Case material has been grouped (n = 132) according to the mean CBF (in grey matter), the difference between groups beeing about 20 ml/100 g/min. Every QEEG profile is the mean polygon from individual polygons belonging to the group. Dashed area = distribution of EEG activity in normals (n = 6) [from *Sulg,* 1969b].

QEEG/rCBF/CMA interdependence. One part of this work, an extensive statistical study on clinical material (144 patients and 6 healthy controls) has been presented as an academic thesis [*Sulg,* 1969b]. The frequency content of the EEG was carefully extracted by means of a especially designed manual period and amplitude analysis [*Sulg,* 1969a]. Despite the heterogeneity of material (patients with different neurologic and psychiatric diagnoses) there were statistically significant correlations between the QEEG and the CBF (fig. 1). Correlation coefficients achieved higher values when the QEEG and CBF measurements were made on the same day ($r = 0.52$, $p < 0.001$) than when the delay was longer than 12 h ($r = 0.48$, $p < 0.01$). In figure 1 it is seen than on pathological slow flow levels there was an increasing shift of EEG activity to the left, i.e. a decrease of alpha activity and increase of activity in slower frequencies. However, the group with the most abundant cortical perfusion is an exception, showing an even

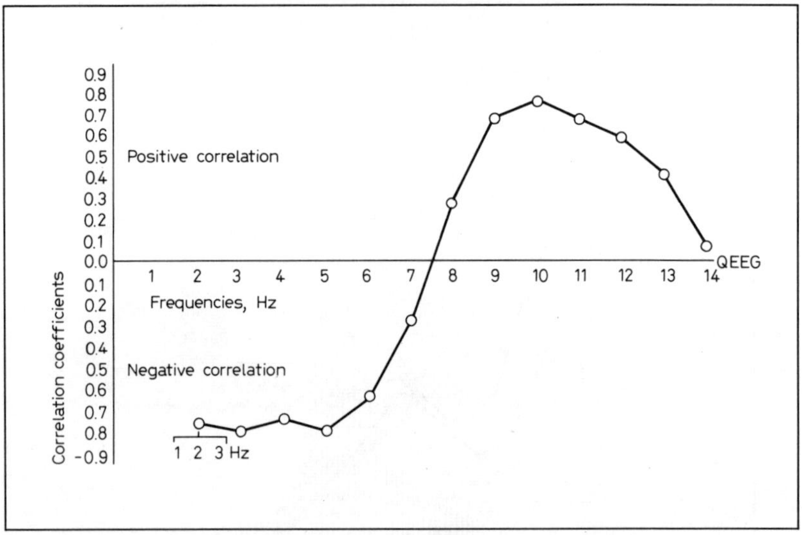

Fig. 2. Correlations between amount of EEG activity in single frequency classes and the mean cortical flow in the same hemisphere. The very first correlation coefficient has been calculated for activity within the 1–3 Hz frequency band. In this material (n = 22) there are only chronic cases without any sign of luxury perfusion [from *Sulg,* 1969b].

more abnormal QEEG profile than the group with the lowest CBF level. This discrepancy is a result of excessive, passive hyperperfusion in severely damaged tissue with dilated nonreactive vessels, the s.c. luxury perfusion syndrome [*Lassen,* 1966]. Furthermore, an unexpected phenomenon is seen in figure 1: all EEG profiles cross each other between 7 and 8 Hz; thus, there is a narrow frequency band without any correlation to the CBF! The same phenomenon of selective indifference appeared when correlation coefficients were calculated separately for every frequency class (fig. 2). It is also seen that interdependence of EEG/CBF decreases toward the higher frequencies. Within the delta frequency range, however, the high level of correlation points to the fact that also slower activity than 1 Hz seems to be correlated negatively to the CBF, and probably also to the CMA. A significant statistical correlation between QEEG and CBF was confirmed in a recent study on brain infarction [*Tolonen* et al., 1981]. Here QEEG parameters derived from 4 different analysis techniques were correlated comparatively to the CBF measured by means of the i.v. method [*Kuikka* et al., 1977]. In stepwise regression analysis, the amount of delta activity derived from the fast Fourier transform (FFT) achieved the highest level of significance ($r = 0.75$, $p < 0.001$).

Reduction and Compression of QEEG Data for EEG Monitoring

Since the EEG is the only brain function which can be recorded and analyzed continuously without active cooperation from monitored subject, it is well suited for brain monitoring in high-risk conditions. A shifting analogue EEG pattern, however, is too tiresome to watch in longer periods. Here computer aid is imperatively needed. A compressed spectral array of power density could be an alternative, but when emphasis lies on easily interpretable display, comprehensible at one glance, then a semicontinuous graph of some few parameters has to be chosen [*Maynard* et al., 1969; *Sulg and Ingvar,* 1970]. There is thus an imperative need for meaningful data reduction. For this end a multivariate regression analysis of 26 different QEEG variables – in relation to the cortical CBF – was performed [*Ingvar and Sulg,* 1969; *Sulg,* 1969b]. From single-frequency bands the 11 Hz achieved the highest significance, but of still higher significance was the frequency corresponding to the mean percentage of the activity polygon, the frequency index (FI). In a later study on 32 mainly psychiatric patients, the FI showed a still stronger correlation ($r = 0.78$, $p < 0.001$) to the metabolic rate of oxygen, $CMRO_2$ [*Ingvar* et al., 1976]. The FI seems thus to be a reliable variable for EEG monitoring. If the FI is derived from zero line-crossing or period analysis, then also the corresponding mean voltage or the energy index [*Sulg,* 1969a] has to be monitored, because just a vanishing frequency/voltage reciprocity has turned out to be a reliable warning sign of danger [*Sulg* et al., 1969].

QEEG in Dysmetabolic Encephalopathies

Quantitative evaluation of EEG in metabolic brain disorders is of value in diagnosis as well as in therapy monitoring. In liver cirrhosis a significant correlation between galactose elimination capacity and the FI has been shown [*Kardel and Stigsby,* 1972]. Trends of the FI usually parallel clinical improvement or impairment [*Rorsman and Sulg,* 1970] or may precede it [*Hawkes* et al., 1970]. Quite similar results were obtained in patients with renal failure [*Hagstam,* 1971]: there was a significant correlation between the degree of azotemia and the FI.

QEEG as a Measure of Brain Dysfunction before and after Open-Heart Surgery

The aim of this study [*Sotaniemi* et al., 1980] was (a) to find some prognostic value of QEEG in surgical treatment, (b) to compare conventional and quantitative EEG interpretation, and (c) to evaluate clinical usefulness of various QEEG methods.

The risk of brain damage in open-heart surgery has been discussed in several papers [*Branthwaite,* 1972; *Seppäläinen,* 1973]. Despite advances in surgical techniques brain damage is reported to occur still quite frequently. In the present study 2 preoperative and 5 postoperative EEG examinations were performed parallel to neurological examination and psychometric testing on 65 patients in a 1-year follow-up study. Also in this study the value of 4 different QEEG methods were evaluated. Following QEEG findings proved to be significant to poor postoperative outcome: (a) slowing of the mean frequency with 2 Hz or more, (b) slowing of alpha mean frequency with 1 Hz or more, and (c) reduction of alpha activity with 30% or more.

Discussion

Despite the evidence discussed above, there are still doubts regarding a close EEG/CGF/CMA interdependence. Indeed, there are also examples which seem to contradict this statemant: by eye opening the CBF does not parallel the increase of EEG frequency content; the slow wave sleep is not accompanied by reduced CMA; in the immature brain the EEG is slow despite higher CBF and CMA than in adults [*Kennedy* et al., 1955]. These contradictions, however, are only illusional: if the eyes open EEG would be analyzed during hypoxia, there would certainly be the same slowing as in the eyes closed EEG. Similarly, the slow immature EEG will become still slower when the CMA would be impaired (e.g. in encephalitis). Thus, a logically identical function mode in all follow-up examinations is a necessary prerequisite for reliable assessment of EEG/CBF/CMA interdependence. Severe brain damage will abolish the coupling of CBF to metabolic autoregulation, but the EEG still reflects adequately the severity of tissue damage [*Sulg,* 1969b]. The peculiar indifference of 7–8 Hz band is probably valid also for EEG/CMA interdependence. It is probably a phenomenon characteristic for organic brain syndrome.

Quantitative studies on QEEG-CMA correlations have hitherto been very limited. Here the emission computed tomography, offering high resolution mapping of regional CMA, wil certainly offer highly interesting information [*Ido* et al., 1981]. Perhaps this novel method will show the way to the hidden key of metabolic code inside the QEEG.

Summary

This paper deals mainly with statistically significant findings from studies on relationships between quantitatively analyzed EEG (QEEG), cerebral blood flow (CBF) and metabolic activity of the brain (CMA).

Frequency content and energy distribution of the EEG are dependent on both CBF and CMA, but closer statistical correlation to the latter points to the fact that the EEG is a bioelectrical paraphenomenon of the CMA. The CBF parallels EEG and CMA trends in pathological conditions only to a certain degree and will be more or less decoupled from this physiological dependence in severe brain damage.

The coupling between EEG and CMA, however, is not so close in statistical terms that it would be possible to calculate the latter from the former, but close enough to help us to understand cerebral disorders with or without concomitant EEG changes. The EEG and its quantitative parameters could thus give us information of prognostic value before or during treatment of metabolic brain disorders. Furthermore, adequately selected QEEG variables can be utilized in continuous brain monitoring, e.g. in high-risk surgery and in intensive care.

References

Branthwaite, M.D.: Neurological damage related to open-heart surgery. Thorax *27:* 748–753 (1972).

Branthwaite, M.D.: Prevention of neurological damage during open-heart surgery. Thorax *30:* 258–261 (1975).

Hagstam, K.E.: EEG frequency content related to chemical blood parameters in chronic uremia. Scand. J. Urolog. Nephrolog. suppl. 7 (1971).

Hjorth, B.: The physical significance of time domain descriptors in EEG analysis. Electroenceph. clin. Neurophysiol. *34:* 321–325 (1973).

Ido, T.; Wan, C.N.; Casella, V.: Labeled 2-deoxy-*D*-glucose, 2-deoxy-2-fluoro-*D*-mannose and 14-C-2-deoxy-2-fluoro-*D*-glucose. J. Label. Comp. Radiopharm. *14:* 175–183 (1978).

Ingvar, D.H.; Sjölund, B.; Ardö, A.: Correlation between dominant EEG frequency, cerebral oxygen uptake und blood flow. Electroenceph. clin. Neurophysiol. *41:* 268–276 (1976).

Ingvar, D.H.; Sulg, I.A.: Regional cerebral blood flow and EEG frequency content in man. Scand. J. clin. Invest. *23:* suppl. 109, pp. 47–66 (1969).

Kennedy, C.; Sokoloff, L.; Anderson, W.; Duffy, P.: Studies in cerebral circulation and metabolism in children. Tr. Am. neurol. Ass. *79:* 196–198 (1955).

Kuikka, J.; Ahonen, A.; Koivula, A.; Kallaranta, T.; Laitinen, J.: An intravenous isotope method for measuring regional cerebral blood flow and volume. Physics Med. Biol. *22:* 958–970 (1977).

Lassen, N.A.: The luxury perfusion syndrome and its possible relation to acute metabolic acidosis localised within the brain. Lancet *ii:* 1113–1115 (1966).

Maynard, D.; Prior, P.F.; Scott, D.F.: Device for continuous monitoring of cerebral activity in resuscitated pateitns. Br. med. J. *iv:* 545–546 (1969).

Obrist, W.D.; Sokoloff, L.; Lassen, N.A.; Lane, M.H.; Butler, R.N.; Feinberg, I.: Relation of EEG to cerebral blood flow and metabolism in old age. Electroenceph. clin. Neurophysiol. *15:* 610–619 (1963).

Obrist, W.D.; Thompson, H.K.; Wang, H.S.; Wilkinson, W.E.: Regional cerebral blood flow estimated by ^{133}Xenon inhalation. Stroke *6:* 245–256 (1975).

Rorsman, G.; Sulg, I.A.: Lactulose treatment of chronic hepatoportal encephalopathy. Acta med. scand. *187:* 337–346 (1970).

Seppäläinen, A.-M.: An EEG follow-up study of cardiac surgery patients; thesis, Helsinki (1973).

Sotaniemi, K.A.; Sulg, I.A.; Hokkanen, T.E.: Quantitative EEG as a measure of cerebral dysfunction before and after open-heart surgery. A part of academical thesis. Electronenceph. clin. Neurophysiol. *50:* 81–95 (1980).

Stigsby, B.; Obrist, W.D.; Sulg, I.A.: Automatic data acquisition and period-amplitude analysis of the EEG. Comput. Progr. Biomed. *3:* 93–104 (1973).

Sulg, I.A.: Manual EEG analysis. Acta neurol. scand. *26:* 31–56 (1969a).

Sulg, I.A.: The quantitated EEG as a measure of brain dysfunction. Scand. J. clin. Invest. *23:* suppl. pp. 1–110 (1969b).

Sulg, I.A.; Ingvar, D.H.: Data reduction in EEG monitoring. Proc. Annu. Meet. Aerospace Med. Ass., St. Louis (1970), pp. 27–32.

Sulg, I.A.; Lindgren, G.; Stigsby, B.: Statistical evaluation of EEG data derived by period- and amplitude analysis. A computer study. Comput. Progr. Biomed. *1:* 20–31 (1969).

Tolonen, U.; Sulg, I.A.: Comparison of quantitative EEG parameters from four different analysis techniques in evaluation of relationships between EEG and CBF in brain infarction. A part of academical thesis. Electroenceph. clin. Neurophysiol. *51:* 177–185 (1981).

I.A. Sulg, MD, Department of Neurology and Clinical Neurophysiology,
University Central Hospital, Oulu (Finland)

Adv. biol. Psychiat., vol. 6, pp. 109–116 (Karger, Basel 1981)

Regional Cerebral Blood Flow in Organic Dementia and Affective Disorders

Lars Gustafson, Jarl Risberg, Peter Silfverskiöld
Department of Psychiatry I, University Hospital, Lund, Sweden

Introduction

There is an urgent need for diagnostic tools which can be used for differential diagnosis of the various types of organic dementias as well as the differentiation between these and normal ageing and pseudo-dementia secondary to psychiatric illness.

The functional activity of the brain has a close coupling to the cerebral oxygen consumption and to cerebral blood flow [*Raichle* et al., 1976]. With the ^{133}Xe clearance technique [*Lassen and Ingvar,* 1963] it became possible to measure the regional cerebral blood flow (rCBF) and thereby the distribution of activity in the cerebral cortex. The principle of this technique is the external recording of the washout of the radioactive tracer ^{133}Xe which is injected into the carotid artery. The development of the ^{133}Xe inhalation technique gave rCBF measurements a wider clinical applicability [*Mallett and Veall,* 1963; *Obrist* et al., 1967; *Risberg,* 1980]. The present paper will review some recent findings from our research in Lund on patients with organic dementia, depression and manic states.

Materials

Organic Dementia

Patients from a prospective study of presenile dementia [*Gustafson,* 1975]. This material of about 100 cases does not include patients with chronic psychoses, oligophrenia, addiction, pre-existing epilepsy, severe somatic disorders or apoplexy with severe neurological defects. The neuropathological findings [*Brun and Gustafson,* 1978] have shown that the presenile dementia group contains mainly cases of Alzheimer's disease (AD), multi-infarct dementia (MID) and Pick's disease (PD) but also a few cases with Jacob-Creutzfeldt's disease.

Affective Disorders

Mania. A group of 26 manic patients with a mean age of 48 years (range 22–80 years) reported recently by *Silfverskiöld* et al. [1980] was studied.

Depression. 46 depressed patients referred to ECT were included. The mean age was 62 years (range 36–83 years). The criteria for selection have been presented elsewhere [*Silfverskiöld* et al., 1981].

Patients with chronic psychoses, addiction, manifest dementia or neurological defects were excluded from the affective groups.

Methods

The psychiatric evaluation and clinical diagnosis were based on formalized rating scales [*Gustafson,* 1975; *Gustafson and Nilsson,* 1981; *Silfverskiöld* et al., 1981]. The AD scale contained clinical features, such as slow progression, spatial disorientation, aphasia, apraxia, agnosia and increased muscular tension. The PD scale contained symptoms, such as personality deterioration, severe confabulation, echolalia, mutism and amimia. The diagnosis of MID was based on the ischaemic score [*Hachinski* et al., 1975].

The rCBF Measurement. The ^{133}Xe inhalation technique in its present form has been used in our laboratory since 1975. The isotope, ^{133}Xe, is inhaled by the patient. 1 min of inhalation of ^{133}Xe mixed with air is followed by 10 min of normal air breathing. The elimination of the tracer is measured simultaneously over 16 areas of each hemisphere by scintillation detectors. The measurement data are computer analyzed and different rCBF parameters are calculated. The initial slope index (ISI) is a reliable flow parameter indicating blood flow in the grey matter [*Risberg* et al., 1975; *Risberg,* 1980]. RCBF can also be measured repeatedly during rest, mental activation and treatment [*Prohovnik* et al., 1980; *Risberg,* 1980].

Results

Organic Dementia

By the standardized clinical evaluation 53 of 65 patients with pre-senile dementia were diagnosed as AD (22 cases) as MID (24 cases) or as PD (7 cases). The remaining 12 cases belonged to a mixed diagnostic group. The mean hemispheric flow values of the three dementia groups [*Gustafson and Risberg,* 1979], a group of 19 non-demented depressed patients [*Johanson* et al., 1979] and a reference group of 22 normal subjects [*Prohovnik* et al., 1980] are presented on table I.

The average flow values of AD, PD and MID cases are significantly lower ($p < 0.001$, t-test for uncorrelated means) than those of depressive and normals. Moreover, AD and PD differed from MID at the 5% level of significance. The most marked group differences were, however, found in the regional distribution of flow values [*Gustafson and Risberg,* 1979]. 19 of the 22 AD cases showed

Table I. Mean hemispheric flow values (ISI) in patients with AD, PD, MID and depression and normal subjects

Diagnose	n	Age	ISI rigth	ISI left	$apCO_2$ mm Hg
AD	22	66.0 ± 6	33.0 ± 6.5	32.4 ± 6.2	37.9 ± 3.6
PD	7	68.0 ± 5	32.9 ± 3.0	32.4 ± 3.9	34.6 ± 1.4
MID	24	65.0 ± 5	32.2 ± 6.7	36.6 ± 6.1	36.5 ± 3.8
Depressed	19	60.0 ± 14	47.0 ± 6.8	47.1 ± 7.0	38.8 ± 3.4
Normals	22	28.0 ± 7.3	53.8 ± 6.3	53.4 ± 6.2	42.7 ± 1.8

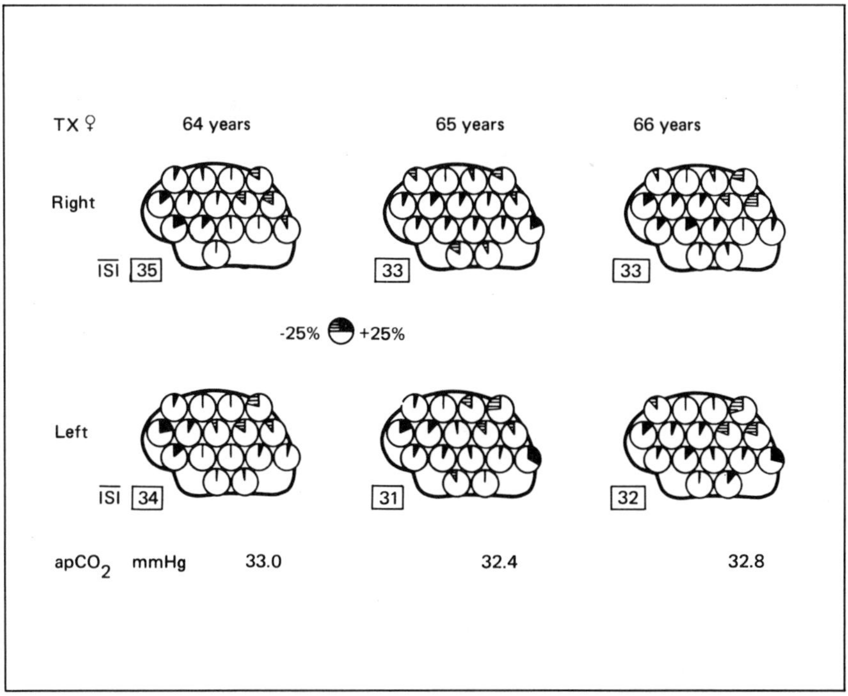

Fig. 1. Repeated rCBF measurements in AD. The mean hemispheric flow values are shown in the boxes. The regional deviations are indicated by the clock symbols in the circles. Black indicates a value above, striped a value below the hemispheric average. A 25% deviation from the mean is equal to 90° in the clock symbol. 12 o'clock indicates a regional value = hemispheric mean. The first rCBF measurement shows a general flow decrease and the typical post-central accentuation of AD. At the second and third measurement an additional flow decrease is observed.

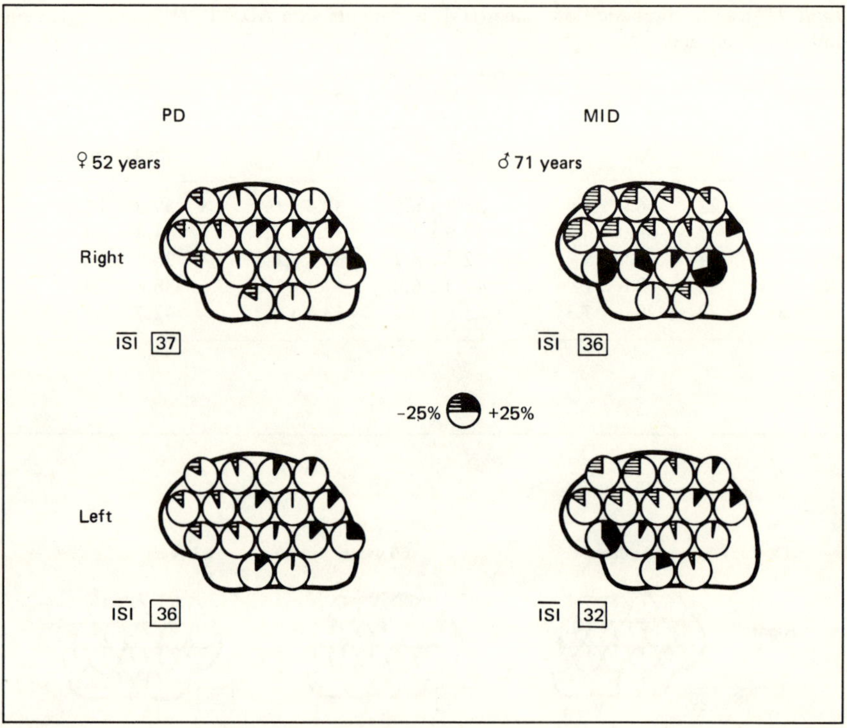

Fig. 2. RCBF in patients with PD and MID.

marked post-central accentuation of the general flow decrease, especially in the parietal lobe. 2 cases in the late stages of the disease had additional frontal flow decreases. Figure 1 shows rCBF values from repeated measurements in a case of AD. The patient showed a slowly progressive dementia with aphasia, agnosia and apraxia.

In patients diagnosed as PD the flow abnormalities were found in frontal regions in 5 out of 7 cases. 1 case had a global flow decrease and 1 showed normal rBCF results. In patients with the tentative diagnosis of MID, 10 cases showed regional and/or global hemispheric right-left asymmetries as shown in figure 2. 5 cases showed a global CBF decrease with no regional abnormalities and 8 cases showed normal rCBF levels and patterns. 1 patient showed a flow pattern of the AD type.

The PD case (Fig. 2) suffered a progressive deterioration with personality change, apathy, euphoria, lack of insight, expressive aphasia and dysgraphia, while orientation and memory were less affected. The MID case had a history of attacks of brain ischaemia, confusional episodes and a mental deterioration with a fluctuating course. Post-mortem investigation confirmed the tentative diagnosis of MID.

Comments. The results indicate that rCBF can be used not only for differentiation between organic dementia and depressive states but also for identification of various types of dementia, such as AD, MID and PD. In the AD and PD groups there was a close correlation between the rCBF and the clinical picture. The flow patterns are in good agreement with the neuropathological findings in AD and PD. In AD the post-central cortical areas are more involved and in PD the frontal and anterio-temporal regions are more affected by the brain disease [*Brun and Gustafson,* 1978]. The brain lesions in MID are more heterogeneous which is in agreement with a less consistent and more fluctuating clinical picture in these cases. In more advanced stages of MID the bi-lateral rCBF measurements show, however, flow asymmetries which are clearly different from the generally symmetric changes in AD and PD. The rCBF method is less sensitive to small and/or deep infarcts. Our findings with the xenon inhalation method are in good agreement with measurements with the ^{133}Xe intra-arterial method in organic dementia. It has been shown that the type and degree of cognitive dysfunction [*Hagberg and Ingvar,* 1976] and the symptom pattern in dementia correlate significantly with the rCBF values [*Gustafson and Risberg,* 1974]. Also the diagnosis and neuropathological findings in deceased cases correlate with previous rCBF values [*Gustafson* et al., 1977].

Affective Disorders

The results in table I show that rCBF in non-demented depressive patients deviates significantly from that of demented patients and normals. The regional flow patterns of patient groups with manic and depressive disorders are shown in figure 3.

The normal subjects had symmetrical flow values which were 5–15% above the hemispheric mean in the frontal lobes and 5–15% below the hemispheric mean in the parietal and occipital regions. This relative hyperfrontality was also found in the manic and depressed groups. The hemispheric mean flow values of the 26 manic patients were, however, significantly lower than those of normals and depressives (t-test, $p < 0.001$). Also the flow values of the larger group of depressed patients ($n = 46$) were significantly lower than those of the normal group. The rCBF differences between manic and depressed patients were still significant when age matched patient groups were compared.

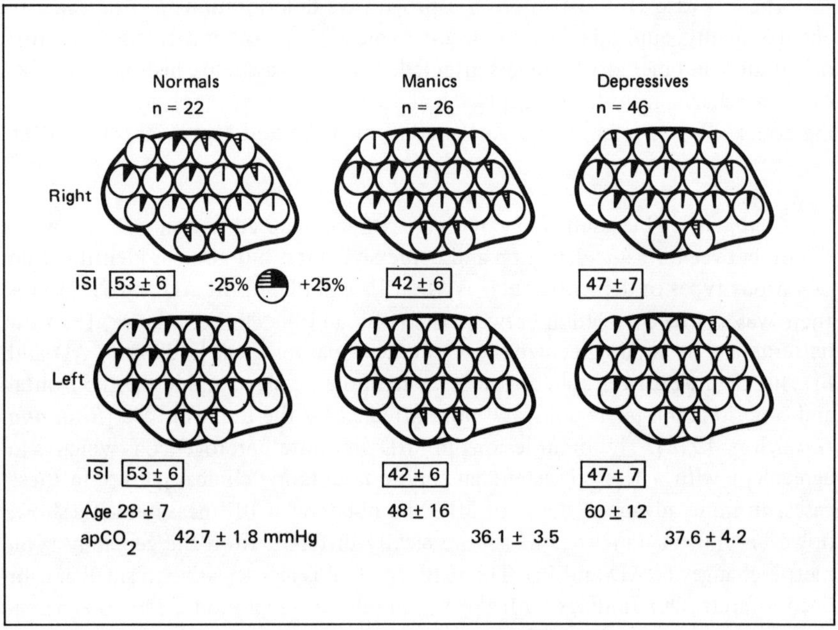

Fig. 3. RCBF in normal subjects and in affective disorders.

Comments. The important question is whether the observed flow differences are related to the mental disorder per se or have some other cause. There are several possible explanations for the lower flow level in manic patients. First this group was on medication with lithium and/or neuroleptics. Neuroleptics have been shown to reduce rCBF especially in frontal areas in paranoid psychoses [*Nilsson* et al., 1977]. We have so far too few measurements on manic patients without medication. 10 manic patients who were re-examined after clinical improvement but on a stable medication showed, however, unchanged low flow values, which might indicate the importance of medication rather than that of clinical changes of the flow level. When differences in age and $apCO_2$ are compensated for, the flow differences between manics, depressives and normals become uncertain. Our rCBF findings do not support the conclusion drawn by *Mathew* et al. [1980] that depressed patients have subnormal flow values. The present findings on hemispheric mean flow values do not, however, exclude that further analyses might show significant relationship between regional flow changes in one or both hemispheres and affective disorders. Results from a study on the effects of ECT in depressed patients have been presented recently [*Silfverskiöld et al.*, 1979].

Summary

With the ^{133}Xe inhalation technique it is possible to measure the functional activity of different cortical areas in both hemispheres simultaneously. This review presents rCBF findings with this technique in presenile dementias and affective disorders. The mean hemispheric flow level is significantly lower in dementia than in normals and depressed patients. In patients with Alzheimer's disease and Pick's disease the most marked flow reduction is found in post- and precentral cortical areas, respectively corresponding to the distribution of cortical degeneration. In multi-infarct dementia focal or global hemispheric right-left asymmetries or a general flow decrease is found. In depressed patients the rCBF level and distribution are normal. The significantly decreased flow level in manic patients might be caused to an important degree by the medical treatment in these patients.

Acknowledgements

We wish to thank Mrs *Maj Lantz* for skillful secretarial aid. The study was supported by the Swedish Medical Research Council (projects 21P-5144, 21X-3950 and 21X-04969), the Swedish Council for Social Science Research and the Swedish Work Environment Fund.

References

Brun, A.; Gustafson, L.: Limbic lobe involvement in presenile dementia. Arch. Psychiat. Nerv. Krankh. *226:* 79–93 (1978).

Gustafson, L.: Psychiatric symptoms in dementia with onset in the presenile period. Acta psychiat. scand. *257:* suppl., pp. 8–35 (1975).

Gustafson, L.; Brun, A.; Ingvar, D.H.: Presenile dementia: clinical symptoms, pathoanatomical findings and cerebral blood flow; in Meyer, Lechner, Reivich, Cerebral vascular disease, pp. 5–9 (Excerpta Medica, Amsterdam/Oxford 1977).

Gustafson, L.; Nilsson, L.: Differential diagnosis of presenile dementia (in press, 1981).

Gustafson, L.; Risberg, J.: Regional cerebral blood flow measurements by the ^{133}Xe inhalation technique in differential diagnosis of dementia. Acta neurol. scand. *60:* suppl. 72, pp. 546–547 (1979).

Hachinski, V.C.; Iliff, L.D.; Zilhka, E.; Boulay, G.H. du; McAllister, V.L.; Marshall, J.; Ross Russell, R.W.; Symon, L.: Cerebral blood flow in dementia. Archs Neurol. Chicago *32:* 632–637 (1975).

Hagberg, B.; Ingvar, D.H.: Cognitive reduction in presenile dementia related to regional abnormalities of the cerebral blood flow. Br. J. Psychiat. *128:* 209–222 (1976).

Johanson, M.; Risberg, J.; Silfverskiöld, P.; Gustafson, L.: Regional cerebral blood flow related to acute memory disturbance following electroconvulsive therapy in depression. Acta neurol. scand. *60:* suppl. 72, pp. 534–535 (1979).

Lassen, N.A.; Ingvar, D.H.: Regional cerebral blood flow measurements in man. Archs Neurol., Chicago *9:* 615–622 (1963).

Mallett, B.L.; Veall, N.: Investigation of cerebral blood flow in hypertension, using radioactive xenon inhalation and extracranial recording. Lancet *i:* 1081 (1963).

Mathew, R.J.; Meyer, J.S.; Semchuk, K.M.; Francis, D.J.; Mortel, K.; Claghorn, J.L.: Cerebral blood flow in depression. Lancet *i:* 1308 (1980).

Nilsson, A.; Risberg, J.; Johanson, M.; Gustafson, L.: Regional changes of cerebral blood flow during haloperidol therapy in patients with paranoid symptoms. Acta neurol. scand. *56:* suppl. 64, pp. 478–479 (1977).

Obrist, W.D.; Thompson, H.K.; King, C.D.; Wang, H.W.: Determination of regional cerebral blood flow by inhalation of ^{133}xenon. Circulation Res. *20:* 124–135 (1967).

Prohovnik, I.; Håkansson, K.; Risberg, J.: Observations on the functional significance of regional cerebral blood flow in 'resting' normal subjects. Neuropsychologia *18:* 203–217 (1980).

Raichle, M.E.; Grubb, R.L.; Gado, M.H.; Eichling, J.O.; Ter-Pogossian, M.T.: Correlation between regional cerebral blood flow and oxidative metabolism. Archs Neurol., Chicago *8:* 523–526 (1976).

Risberg, J.: Regional cerebral blood flow measurements by ^{133}Xe inhalation: methodology and applications in neuropsychology and psychiatry. Brain Language *9:* 9–34 (1980).

Risberg, J.; Ali, Z.; Wilson, E.M.; Wills, E.L.; Halsey, J.H.: Regional cerebral blood flow by ^{133}xenon inhalation. Preliminary evaluation of an initial slope index in patients with unstable flow compartments. Stroke *6:* 142–148 (1975).

Silfverskiöld, P.; Gustafson, L.; Johanson, M.; Risberg, J.: Regional cerebral blood flow related to the effect of electroconvulsive therapy in depression; in Obiols, Ballús, Gonzalez Monclús, Pujol, Biological psychiatry today (Elsevier/North-Holland Biomedical Press, Amsterdam 1979).

Silverskiöld, P.; Gustafson, L.; Johanson, M.; Risberg, J.: Regional cerebral blood flow in affective disorders. 12th CINP Congress, Gothenburg, in press, 1981.

L. Gustafson, MD, Department of Psychiatry I, University Hospital,
S-22185 Lund (Sweden)

Adv. biol. Psychiat., vol. 6, pp. 117–120 (Karger, Basel 1981)

Habituation of Alpha Rhythm Blocking in Structured Neuroses

G. Iorio, R. Tissot

Clinica Psichiatrica, Prima Facoltà di Medicina e Chirurgia, Università di Napoli, Napoli, Italia; Clinique Psychiatrique de Bel-Air, Chêne-Bourg, Genève, Suisse

The present study on the habituation of alpha rhythm blocking to visual stimuli is a part of a long-term research program, still in progress at the Psychiatric Clinic of the University of Geneva, concerned with assimilation/accommodation balance in hysterical and obsessive patients.

In his work about cognitive development, *Piaget* emphasizes the role of the *adjustment* that characterizes every living being and assumes various forms or structures according to their development stage. The adjustment process shows two opposite and complementary aspects: the *assimilation,* i.e. the integration of external elements or events to the subject's structures, and the *accommodation,* i.e. the transformation of these structures depending on the external changes of the environment.

Piaget introduces the concept of 'balance' in order to explain the mechanism that undeline the interaction between the subject and his environment. The mental adjustment is considered as an extension of the biological adjustment; it is the form of superior balance that leads to an adequate construction of the knowledge and of the action. An imbalance between the two aspects of adjustment will lead, therefore, to a *preeminence* of assimilation or accommodation.

In the thinking processes with preeminence of assimilation, the logic-mathematical constructions prevail over the properties of the external objects. The observable data are preferably attributed to the central mechanisms of the subject's action and explained by means of these mechanisms, and therefore by the internal coordination of the logical reasoning; the physical causality is only a reflexetion of the logical causality that, therefore, may be more or less adequate.

In the case of the accommodation preeminence, the subject's processes are, in a way, 'delegated' to the objects; the observable data are mainly attributed to the intrinsic properties of the external objects. If they are excessively accommodated to the pecularities of the objects, the 'delegated' processes will be insufficiently coordinated among themselves. As a consequence, the assimilation preeminence promotes the awareness of the contradictions arising from the coordination of both reasoning and action. Conversely, the accomodation preeminence will preferably bring to the awareness of the contradictions concerned with external objects.

The lack of balance between assimilation and accommodation could explain either a particular way of being in front of reality, or the choice of one symptom in a distress situation: in this case, the assimilation preeminence could promote the development of hysterical neuroses. The assimilator subject is inclined to emphasize the aspects or the properties of external objects according to his own logical processes; therefore, in a confluctual or uncontrollable situation dominated by distress, he will be able only to lay the blame on himself, that is to say on his body, which is for him, finally, the instrument of any cause.

On the contrary, a lack of balance tending toward the accommodation preminence could determine the development of obsessive neuroses. In the same conflictual and distressing situations, the subject who is inclined to adjust too much his own logical processes to the peculiarities of the external objects will incessantly verify the efficacy of actions and perceptions that he is not able to control. The control of external reality escapes him, because the legality of the universal causality is immanent to the external objects and he is not able to integrate it to his logical processes.

If we consider the alpha-blocking rhythm mainly as an expression of the accommodation process of the subject's structures to the external stimuli, we can expect that subjects with assimilation preeminence (and among them are the hysterical patients) will show few modifications of their cerebral electrical activity under the influence of external stimuli, that is to say that they will rapidly habituate themselves to them.

Furthermore, the assimilation preeminence should facilitate the control of the subject's structure modifications induced by external stimuli and particularly the control of the alpha rhythm by biofeedback. On the contrary, in the subjects dominated by the accommodation preeminence (and among them are the obsessives), the modifications of the subject's structures depending on the object or on the external stimuli prevail. This could explain why obsessives or accommodator subjects have a lower habituation rate. In this case, since the external properties of the object prevail over the mental logical processes, any attempt to control the accommodation to the properties of the external world, as well as of the alpha rhythm by means of biofeedback, should fail.

Methods

To verify this hypothesis, we used some classical antinomies, two tests of genetic psychology, a test of accommodation of the action to the visual data and a neurophysiological test: the habituation of the alpha rhythm blocking to visual flashes with or without auditive biofeedback control.

We applied the above-mentioned test battery to seven control subjects (colleagues, a psychologist and secretaries) and to 9 patients, 4 of them affected by hysteria (hemiplegia, alexia, syncopes, amnesia) and 5 suffering from classical phobic-obsessive neuroses.

The habituation of alpha blocking to light stimuli with closed eyes has been observed in two different situations, namely with and without auditive control (biofeedback).

The EEG was recorded from two symmetrical occipital leads. During the recording, the subjects received 250 flashes with a frequency of $^{1}]_{3}$ s. A slight auditive stimulus was given if the tracing showed any evidence of alertness lowering. After a short interval, a second series of 250 flashes was given, with an auditive control by means of a sound sent through a casing and modulated by the alpha rhythm of the subjects. The absence of the alpha rhythm produced the sound; thus blocking of the alpha rhythm after a flash produced a sound which the subjects were requested to inhibit. In this way, they could control their own habituation to the flash-induced alpha blocking.

The blocking was visually evaluated on the EEG tracing: a complete alpha blocking was rated as 1, a partial blockings as $^{1}/_{2}$ and the absence of any blocking as 0. Blocks of 5 consecutive reactions were evaluated, so that each session was described by 50 values varying from 0 to 5.

The first of ten consecutive flashes without a blocking reaction was considered as the beginning of habituation. Some subjects did not show any habituation even after 250 stimuli, which was the programmed limit. This makes difficult the evaluation of the modifications induced by the auditive control on the habituation phenomenon in these subjects.

For furhter evaluation, we did not consider the habituation curves themselves, but the areas under the curves, and we determined the effect of the auditive control as the percentage of modification of the habituation area under auditive biofeedbaack with respect to the habituation area without auditive biofeedback.

Results

The assimilator subjects habituated more rapidly than the accommodators ($p < 0.01$). The same results were found in hysterical subjects compared to obsessives ($p < 0.05$). For all subjects, this rate of habituation was correlated with the coefficient assimilation/accommodation calculated from the results of psychological tests ($r = 0.629$, $p < 0.05$). The auditive control of alpha blocking produced an increase of the habituation ability in assimilators, while it reduced it in accommodators ($p < 0.025$). Hysterics showed the same trend as assimilators; conversely, the obsessives had the same characteristics as the accommodators. However, because of the high individual variability, the difference between hysterics and obsessives in habituation rate under auditive control was not significant. The modifications of habituation under the effect of auditive control were correlated with the coefficient assimilation/accommodation ($r = -0.527$, $p < 0.05$; table I).

Table I. Habituation – Assimilation – Accomodation Differences between Hysterics and Obsessives

Subjects	(1) Assimilation / accomodation coefficient	(2) Stimulation habituation	(3) Habituation Gain by means of bio feedback
Assimilator controls + hysterics (7)	– 1.20 ± 0.47 $p < 0.05$	134.4 ± 17.8 $p < 0.01$	+ 41.4 ± 31.9 $p < 0.025$
Accommodator controls + obsessives (8)	+ 1.51 ± 0.52	197.6 ± 46.3	– 11.6 ± 44.3
Hysterics (4)	– 1.27 ± 0.63 $p < 0.05$	132.6 ± 21.8 $p < 0.05$	+ 24.7 ± 32.3 n.s.
Obsessives (5)	+ 1.76 ± 0.34	209.4 ± 55.6	– 4.8 ± 42.2
Correlation coefficient to (1)		R = 0.629 $p < 0.05$	R = 0.527 $p < 0.05$

Conclusions

Taken together, the results of psychological testing of habituation recording and habituation modification in a situation of biofeedback indicate that: (1) the reflective way of thinking of the hysterics is dominated by the preeminence of assimilation; (2) the reflective way of thinking of the obsessives is dominated by the preeminence of accommodation; (3) the preeminence of assimilation is associated to a good ability of perceptive delegation and to a good ability of habituation, which is well controlled in a biofeedback situation; (4) the preeminence of accommodation is associated to a weak ability of perceptive delegation and to a weak ability of habituation, scarcely controllable by means of a biofeedback; (5) the coefficient assimilation/accommodation in all the sujects (controls and patients) is correlated with their habituation ability and with their ability to control the habituation phenomenon by means of a biofeedback.

These results support our original hypothesis, that the reflective thought of the hysterics is mainly assimilative and that this feature is correlated with their habituation and biofeedback control ability; on the other hand, they do not allow us to assert that the symptom choice in these classical neuroses depends on the assimilative or accommodative character of thought. In this way, our results represent a preliminary experimental verification of a research hypothesis worth further investigation.

G. Iorio, MD, Clinica Psichatrica, Prima Facoltà di Medicina e Chirurgia,
Università di Napoli, I-80125 Napoli (Italy)

Adv. biol. Psychiat., vol. 6, pp. 121–125 (Karger, Basel 1981)

Do Psychoactive Drugs Affect the EEG from the Cerebral Hemispheres Differently?

Peter Irwin, Max Fink

Department of Psychiatry and Behavioral Science, School of Medicine, SUNY at Stony Brook, N.Y. and the Long Island Research Institute, Stony Brook, N.Y., USA

Quantitative electroencephalography (EEG) is useful in phase-I pharmacologic studies to identify and classify psychoactive drugs and to define their pharmacodynamic properties [*Fink,* 1969; *Itil,* 1974]. The left occipital to vertex derivation is usually selected for spectral analysis. A spectral profile is developed by comparing a drug's effects to those of placebo. Classification is based on the similarity of this profile to that of established psychoactive compounds. Drugs sharing the same EEG profile have therapeutic value in the same psychiatric populations [*Fink,* 1969, 1978]. Reports that hemispheric localization of function may extend to mood and cognition and that the pathophysiology of schizophrenia and depression may be hemisphere-specific [*Wexler,* 1980] led us to question whether psychoactive drugs affect the cerebral hemispheres differently.

After bilateral electroconvulsive therapy, increases in EEG slowing [*Abrams* et al., 1970] and variability of the amplitudes within a patient's records [*d'Elia and Perris,* 1973, 1974] are more pronounced in the left hemisphere. Neuroleptics affect the hemispheres variably [*Serafetinides,* 1973; *d'Elia* et al., 1977]. Voltage is reported to be higher on the left side with chlorpromazine and clopenthixol, but higher on the right side with penfluridol and thiothixene. No hemispheric differences were found with haloperidol or molindone. In extensive studies, *Goldstein and Stoltzfus* [1973] reported that *d*-amphetamine and chlorpromazine reduced hemispheric EEG amplitude differences, cannabis increased the differences, hallucinogens D-675 and LSD-25 reversed the right/left ratio, and sedatives, minor tranquilizers, and placebo produced no change.

We have investigated lateral differences in response to drugs of different classes using power spectral density analysis of the resting EEG. In this report, we ask whether the profile, time course, or magnitude of EEG change in response to different substances differs between derivations from each side of the head, and whether there is a relationship to cerebral dominance.

Methods

Drugs. We examined the EEG records from single-dose studies of five psychoactive compounds: phenytoin (1 g, n = 12); haloperidol (4 mg, n = 10); diphenhydramine (50 mg, n = 18); imipramine (30 mg, n = 11); and mianserin (10 mg, n = 11). Each was administered orally in a placebo-controlled, balanced order, cross-over design. Doses were selected in pilot studies both for their CNS activity and their tolerability by all subjects. EEGs were sampled in 15-min segments at half-hourly or hourly intervals up to 7.5 hours post-drug. Descriptions of the methods and findings are published elsewhere [*Fink and Irwin,* 1979, 1980; *Fink* et al., 1977, 1979].

Statistics. Percent of spectral intensity per Hz was combined into 2-Hz bands up to 17 Hz and into 4-Hz bands between 18 and 29 Hz. Other variables were average frequency and total intensity, and average absolute difference per Hz between two spectra (baseline and post-drug, left and right hemispheres). Hemispheric interrelationships were examined in 11 left/right ratios: total intensity and its standard deviation, mean frequency, and intensity in bands 0–3, 4–7, 8–13, and 14–20 Hz (in units of both μV^2 and percentage of total). Differences between drug and placebo and between hemispheres were identified using a repeated measures analysis of covariance for each EEG variable separately. Results were corroborated by analysis of variance of post-drug minus baseline differences.

Results

Lateral Activity. Spectral profiles for phenytoin, diphenhydramine, and mianserin were well-defined. Patterns of drug-induced change in the right hemisphere (O_2–C_z) were found to be identical to those in the left (O_1–C_z). They differed only in the level of probability of the discrimination from placebo in some bands. At the times of peak effect, the direction of significant changes in all bands was the same for both derivations.

The profiles for imipramine and haloperidol were not well-defined at these doses. Discomfort in some subjects at higher doses limited the dose selected for study, and for many subjects the dosages were below the measurement threshold. Neither derivation was superior in identifying the activity of these drugs (table I).

The time course of EEG effects for all drugs was indistinguishable between the hemispheres.

Hemispheric Interrelationship. After mianserin, left/right ratios were reduced in 4–7 Hz percent intensity, increased in 8–13 Hz, and increased in mean frequency. Changes from baseline were greater in the right hemisphere than in the left. Other left/right ratios did not show a drug-placebo difference. Spectral differences between derivations were reduced from baseline differences by diphenhydramine and mianserin, but unchanged by other drugs, relative to placebo.

Table I. Spectral profiles of differences from placebo at O_1-C_z and O_2-O_z derivations, based on analyses of covariance (ANCOVA). Profiles differ between drug classes, but are similar for both derivations. Differences are not found between the derivations at the times of peak drug effect

	Phenytion 1,000 mg		Haloperidol 4 mg		Diphenhydramine 50 mg		Imipramine 30 mg		Mianserin 10 mg	
	O_1	O_2	O_1	O_2	O_1	O_2	O_1	O_2	O_1	O_2
Total intensity									– –	– –
Mean frequency	+ +	+ +							– –	– –
Hz % total intensity										
0–1					+ +	+ +			+ +	+ +
2–3	– –	–			+ +	+ +			+ +	+ +
4–5	– –	– –			+ +	+ +			+ +	+ +
6–7	–	– –	+ +	+ +	+ +	+ +			+ +	+ +
8–9					– –	– –			– –	
10–11			–	– –	–	–			– –	– –
12–13					+	+ +				
14–15										+
16–17								+ +		
18–21	+	+ +			+	+ +	+			
22–25		+				+ +			+ +	+ +
26–29	+	+ +			+	+ +			+	+ +

+ +, – – $p < 0.05$
+, – $p < 0.10$
ANCOVA

Functional Relationship. Of the 40 subjects included in these studies, 4 had left hand/left eye preference. While no lateral differences respecting hand or eye preference were found, these 4 subjects had a larger EEG response to drugs than did the other subjects. In each study, one of these subjects had the greatest response of all subjects.

Discussion

For these drugs we find the profiles and, at these intervals of measurement, the time courses of EEG change to be equivalent in the two hemispheres. The compounds include representatives of the antidepressant and antipsychotic classes. Only after mianserin did we observe a hemispheric difference in the magnitute of drug-induced EEG change. This is seen in lateral comparisons of changes between pre-drug and post-drug spectra, in spectral differences between hemispheres at each time of sampling, and in left/right percent intensity ratios.

The lateral asymmetry in drug response seen here, and reported by others, is amplitude-sensitive but is not frequency-specific. The spectral effects of these psychoactive substances are not hemisphere-specific in pattern or in temporal course. The differences in the magnitude of response may have many sources in the signal processing system or in the anatomy and/or physiology of the brain. For pharmaco-EEG assessments, individual differences in biological factors and the lack of rationale in theory or experience make the selection of either hemisphere arbitrary.

For both mianserin and diphyenhydramine, the SDIs indicate that post-drug EEG spectra are more bilaterally symmetrical than at baseline. Since the EEG frequency distribution is so markedly altered by both drugs, it is unclear what these reductions in bilateral spectral differences signify. The sedative symptoms accompanying these EEG changes make the conditions similar to light sleep, where bilateral synchrony of EEG activity is enhanced.

The greatest individual responses to these substances were found among subjects who were left-handed and who preferred their left eye in sighting. Although many functional associations with left-handedness have been documented [*Hardyck and Petrinovich,* 1977; *Herron,* 1980], we are not aware of other studies of behavior-altering interventions in which a differential response of left-handed and/or left eye preferent subjects has been observed. This finding remains of interest.

Summary

We examined the effects of single doses of mianserin, imipramine, haloperidol, phenytoin, and diphenhydramine, on EEG power spectra in normal male volunteers in placebo-controlled, balanced order, cross-over studies designed to determine the EEG profile of each drug. EEG from the left and right occipital-vertex derivations (O_1-C_z, O_2-C_z) was sampled in 15-min segments before and at multiple intervals after drug ingestion.

The band distribution and temporal pattern of changes from baseline were equivalent in the two hemispheres for all drugs. The magnitude of change was greater in the right hemisphere after mianserin, but was not laterally different after the other compounds. Hemispheric asymmetry was reduced after mianserin and diphenhydramine. Left-hand/left-eye dominant subjects showed a greater EEG responsivity to these substances. A single derivation remains adequate for pharmaco-EEG profile assessment.

References

Abrams, R.; Volavka, J.; Roubicek, J.; Dornbush, R.; Fink, M.: Lateralized EEG changes after unilateral and bilateral electroconvulsive therapy. Dis. nerv. Syst. *31:* suppl., pp. 28–33 (1970).

d'Elia, G.; Jacobsson, L.; von Knorring, L.; et al. Changes in psychopathology in relation to EEG variables and visual averaged evoked responses (VAER) in schizophrenic patients treated with penfluridol or thiothixene. Acta psychiat. scand. *55:* 209–318 (1977).

d'Elia, G.; Perris, C.: Cerebral functional dominance and memory functions: an analysis of EEG integrated amplitude in depressive psychotics. Acta psychiat. scand. *255:* suppl., pp. 143–157 (1974).

Fink, M.: EEG and human psychopharmacology. A. Rev. Pharmacol. *9:* 241–258 (1969).

Fink, M.: EEG and psychopharmacology; in Cobb, van Duijn, Contemporary clinical neurophysiology. Electroenceph. clin. Neurophysiol. *45:* suppl. 34, pp. 41–56 (1978).

Fink, M.; Irwin, P.: CNS effects of antihistamines diphenhydramine and terfenadine (RMI 9918). Pharmakopsychiatr. Neuro-Psychopharmakol. *12:* 35–44 (1979).

Fink, M.; Irwin, P.: EEG and behavioral profile of flutroline (CP-36, 584), a novel antipsychotic drug. Psychopharmacology *72:* 67–71 (1980).

Fink, M.; Irwin, P.; Gastpar, M.; DeRidder, J.J.: EEG, blood level, and behavioral effects of the antidepressant mianserin (Org GB-94). Psychopharmacology *54:* 249–254 (1977).

Fink, M.; Irwin, P.; Sannita, W.; Papakostas, Y.; Green, M.A.: Phenytoin: EEG effects and plasma levels in volunteers. Therap. Drug Monit. *1:* 93–100 (1979).

Goldstein, L.; Stoltzfus, N.W.: Psychoactive-drug-induced changes of interhemispheric EEG amplitude relationships. Agents Actions *3:* 124–132 (1973).

Hardyck, C.; Petrinovich, L.F.: Left-handedness. Psychol. Bull. *84:* 385–404 (1977).

Herron, J. (ed.): Neuropsychology of left-handedness (Academic Press, New York 1980).

Itil, T.M.: Quantitative pharmaco-electroencephalography; in Itil, Psychotropic drugs and the human EEG. Mod. Probl. Pharmacopsychiat., vol. 8, pp. 43–75 (Karger, Basel 1974).

Serafetinides, E.A.: Voltage laterality in the EEG of psychiatric patients. Dis. nerv. Syst. *34:* 190–191 (1973).

Wexler, B.E.: Cerebral laterality and psychiatry: a review of the literature. Am. J. Psychiat. *137:* 279–291 (1980).

Max Fink, MD, Department of Psychiatry and Behavioral Sciences,
School of Medicine, Stony Brook, NY 11794 (USA)

Adv. biol. Psychiat., vol. 6, pp. 126–142 (Karger, Basel 1981)

Confirmation of Pharmaco-EEG Predictions Concerning Pharmacodynamic Properties of an Anxiolytic Sedative by Sleep Studies

B. Saletu, J. Grünberger, I. Stöllberger

Section of Pharmacopsychiatry, Psychiatric University Clinic, Vienna, Austria

Introduction

As all-night EEG investigations of the effect of sleep-promoting drugs on the central nervous system (CNS) are difficult to perform and are – moreover – very time-consuming, it seems desirable that the design and planning of such great research efforts is not only based just on animal pharmacology but rather on human pharamcodynamic data as well. The quantitative pharmaco-EEG method has been proven to be a valuable instrument in early clinical drug evaluations in man as it is possible to predict: (1) whether a drug has any effect on the CNS as compared with placebo; (2) to which psychopharmacological class it eventually belongs; (3) at which time, and (4) in which dosage it acts [*Fink,* 1969, *Itil,* 1974; *Saletu,* 1976; *Herrmann* et al., 1979].

Furthermore, the equipotency of an experimental substance to clinically well-known drugs and the equipotency of different galenic formulations of a compound may be determined objectively and quantitatively [*Saletu* et al., 1976; *Saletu,* in press; *Saletu and Taeuber,* 1980]. However, the literature is scarce concerning the relationship of drug-induced changes in brain function recorded in the waking state to that in the sleep state. In recent years we had the opportunity to carry out both pharmaco-EEG trials *and* all-night sleep investigations with one and the same compound, brotizolam (WE 941).

Brotizolam is a new triazolothienodiazepine and chemically a 2-bromo-4-(2-chlorophenyl)-9-methyl-6H-thieno(3,2-f)-1,2-(4-triazolo)(4,3-a)diazepine. The compound shows certain similarities to the 1,4-benzodiazepines, but one annelled ring is replaced by a thiophene ring, while at the same time another heterocyclus is annelled to the 7-membered diazepine ring [*Weber* et al., 1978].

Pharmacological investigations in 8 different animal species showed a marked sedation already after oral dosages of a few mg/kg [Boehringer, Ingelheim 1976]. However, quite in contrast to known tranquilizers and barbiturates, brotizolam administered in high doses does not induce coma but rather sleep. It seems further an interesting anxiolytic sedative, as its half-life is very short (3.6–4.4 h), shows extremenly low toxicity.

Evaluating the encephaloptropic, psychotropic and pharmacodynamic properties of brotizolam by means of quantitative EEG and psychometric analyses, we recently could demonstrate that the drug exerts a significant effect on the CNS [*Saletu* et al., 1979; *Grünberger* et al., 1978]. While in a population of 10 normal subjects the EEG power spectral density analysis demonstrated no changes after placebo, 0.1, 0.3 and 0.5 mg WE 941 and 30 mg flurazepam induced statistically significant alterations characterized by an increase in beta activity, a decrease in alpha activity and increase in average frequency ('anxiolytic pharmaco-EEG profile'). In addition, 0.3 and 0.5 mg WE 941 and 30 mg flurazepam produced a significant augmentation of beta activity indicating hypnotic qualities. Considering spontaneous and placebo-induced alteration, evaluation of the time- and dose-effect relationship indicated that all active substances exerted a tranquilizing effect throughout 8 h, while the hypnotic properties of 0.1 mg WE 941 were minimal (up to the 4th hour), those of 0.3 mg WE 941 were moderate (up to 6 h) and those of 0.5 mg WE 941 were marked (up to 8 h). The WE 941 dosage found to be equipotent to 30 mg flurazepam was between 0.5 and 0.3 mg. Heart rate and blood pressure exhibited no relevant changes, while side effects including fatique, drowsiness and dizziness were mostly observed after 0.5 mg WE 941.

Based on psychometric investigations we too could demonstrate that WE 941 exerts a significant psychoactivity starting in the 2nd hour, peaking in the 4th hour and declining slowly thereafter [*Grünberger* et al., 1978]. We concluded that 0.1 mg WE 941 is the minimal effective psychoactive dosage exerting a tranquilizing effect, while the 0.5-mg dose and to some extent also the 0.3-mg dose induce a sedative effect and thus may be regarded as the hypnotic dosages.

The aim of the present study was to prove these predictions by means of a double-blind, placebo-controlled, all-night sleep EEG investigation involving the evaluation of both objective and subjective sleep and awakening variables.

Material and Methods

10 normal healthy volunteers (5 males and 5 females) in ages ranging from 23 to 35 years (mean 27.8 years), heights from 155 to 192 cm (mean 171.1 cm) and weights from 47 to 80 kg (mean 60.8 kg) were included in the double-blind, placebo-controlled, cross-over study. They were not allowed to take any psychoactive drugs 3 weeks before and/or during the period of the study.

The subjects spent 13 nights in the laboratory: 2 adaptation nights, 1 baseline night, 5 drug nights (0.1, 0.2 and 0.5 mg brotizolam; placebo and 30 mg flurazepam as the reference substance) and 5 wash-out nights. The dose of 0.2 mg was chosen because some pilot studies suggested that already this low dosage of brotizolam may be sleep-inducing. The drugs were orally administered in 3-day intervals in a randomized fashion at bedtime (10.30 p.m.). A written informed consent was obtained.

Polygraphic all-night recordings were carried out between 10.30 p.m. and 6.00 a.m. in two identically shielded rooms (thus, the total sleep recording time was fixed). The electrodes were attached according to the international10/20 system. In addition to the EEG channels C_4-A_1, O_2-A_1 and O_2-Cz, two REM channels and the submental EMG was recorded on an 8-channel R-611 Beckmann polygraph. Four channels (O_2-Cz, EMG and 2 REM) were recorded on a Hewlett-Packard 3968 tape recorder as well. 30-sec epochs were scored according to the criteria of *Rechtschaffen and Kales* [1968].

In the morning the subjects completed (subsequently to the morning toilet and the breakfast) a sleep questionnaire for the subjective evaluation of their quality of sleep and awakening [*Saletu* et al., 1974]. Thereafter, they carried out a series of psychometric tests including the *Grünberger* [1977] AD test ('Alphabetischer Durchstreichtest' = alphabetical cross-out test) for quantification of attention (total score) and concentration (errors in percent of the total score) and attention variability; the *Grünberger* [1977] psychomotor activity ('Feinmotorik') test and tapping for determination of changes in psychomotor activity and drive; reaction time as determined on the 'Wiener Reaktionsgerät'; critical flicker frequency (CFF); after-effect (Archimedean spiral), a 'semantic differential polarity profile' [*Osgood* et al., 1975] for measurement of affectivity; the von Zerssen 'Befindlichkeits-Skala' for quantitative evaluation of mood [*von Zerssen* et al., 1970], and pupillometry.

Statistical analysis included the three-way analysis of variance (Anova), the t-test and the Newman-Keuls test as well as the Friedman's rank Anova, the Wilcoxon and the multiple Wilcoxon test. By such means the changes during each night were compared with the baseline night, and differences between drug-induced changes and placebo-induced alterations and their respective wash-out nights were investigated.

Results

1. Objective Sleep Variables

Intermittent wakefulness *(stage W)* decreased significantly ($p < 0.05–0.01$, Wilcoxon test) after all administered substances as compared with the baseline night, while in wash-out nights no significant changes were observed with one exception of a significant decrease of intermittent wakefulness in the wash-out night after 30 mg flurazepam (fig. 1). However, there were no significant differences between the drug nights and placebo as well as between the drug wash-out nights and the placebo wash-out nights.

Stage 1 demonstrated only after 0.5 mg brotizolam a significant decrease as compared with the baseline night (fig. 2). There was an increase in stage 1 in the wash-out night after 0.1 mg brotizolam. The decrease in stage 1 after 0.5 mg brotizolam was also significant as compared with placebo, as was the attenuation of stage 1 in the wash-out night after 30 mg flurazepam as compared with the placebo wash-out night.

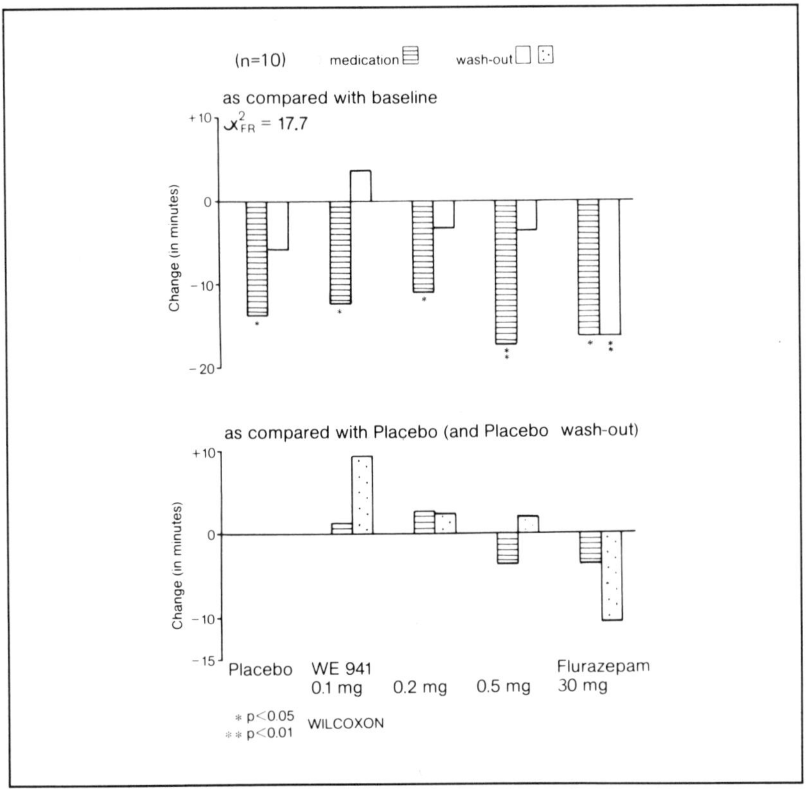

Fig. 1. Changes in stage W (intermittent wakefulness) after single doses of brotizolam, 30 mg flurazepam and placebo. Medication nights and wash-out nights are represented in the abscissa, drug-induced changes (min) as compared with baseline are shown in the upper ordinate, changes as compared with placebo or with the placebo wash-out night are indicated in the lower ordinate. A decrease in intermittent wakefulness can be seen after all administered substances as compared with baseline, while the changes did not reach the level of statistical significance as compared with placebo or the placebo wash-out night, respectively.

Stage 2 demonstrated after all administered substances an increase but significantly so after 0.5 mg brotizolam, 30 mg flurazepam, and placebo as compared with baseline, while the wash-out nights did not show any significant alterations as compared with baseline with the exception of an increase in stage 2 in the wash-out night after 30 mg flurazepam (fig. 3). The latter was also the case if one compares the drug wash-out night with the placebo wash-out night.

Stage 3 and *stage 4* did not show any significant changes as compared with the baseline night, nor as compared with placebo or placebo wash-out night.

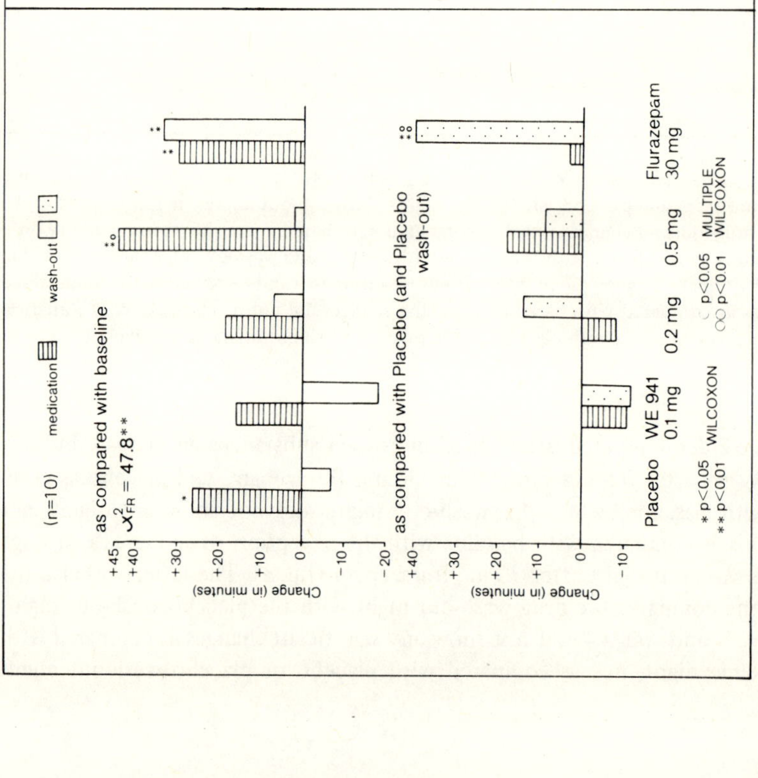

Fig. 2. Changes in stage 1 after single doses of brotizolam, 30 mg flurazepam and placebo.

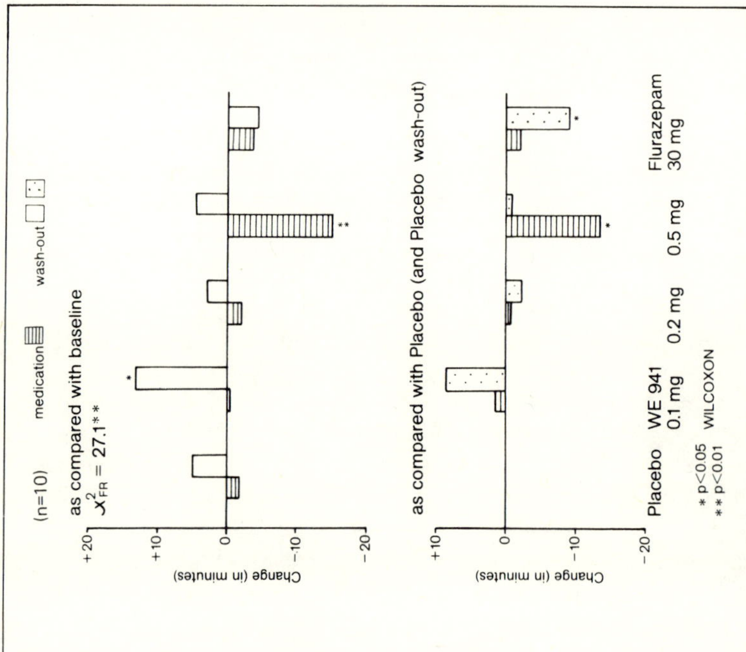

Fig. 3. Changes in stage 2 after single doses of brotizolam, 30 mg flurazepam and placebo.

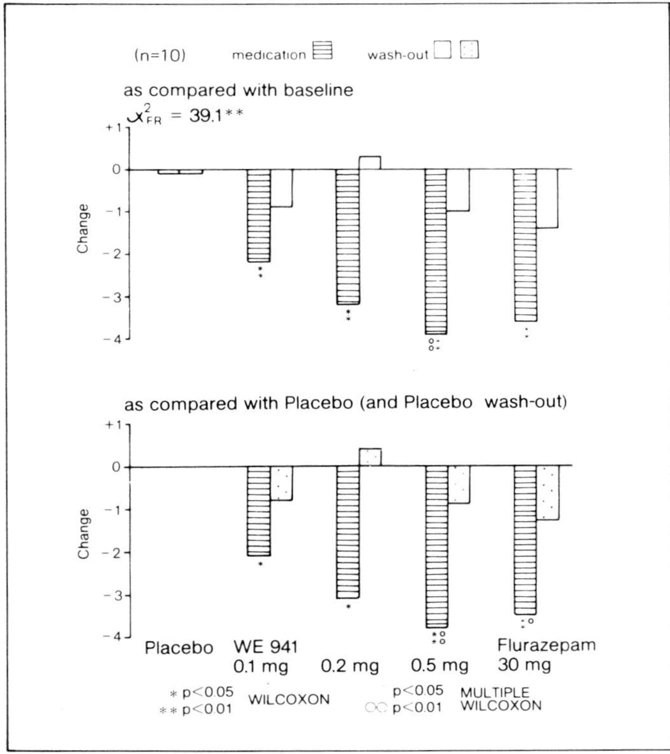

Fig. 4. Changes in stage REM after single oral doses of brotizolam, 30 mg flurazepam and placebo.

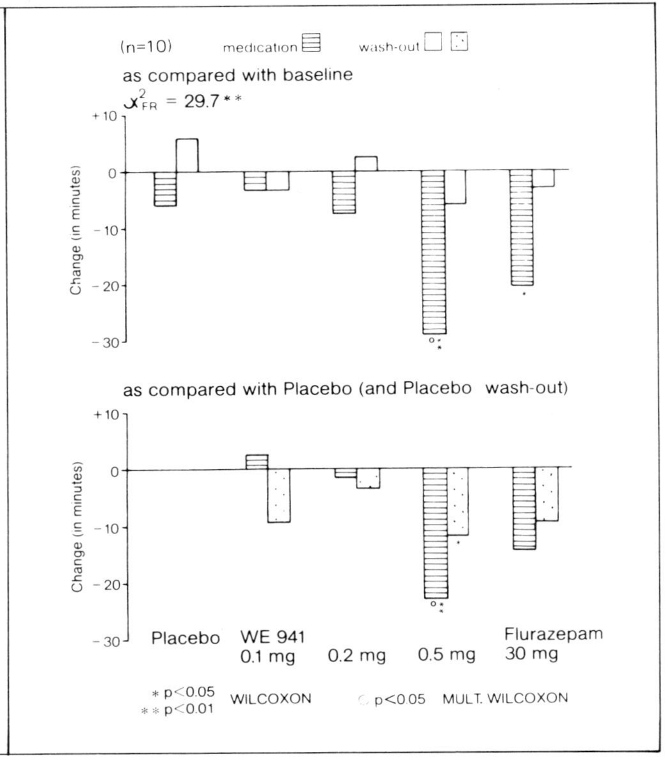

Fig. 5. Changes in the number of wakenings after single doses of brotizolam, 30 mg flurazepam and placebo.

REM stages decreased significantly after 0.5 mg brotizolam and 30 mg flurazepam as compared with the baseline night (fig. 4). The reduction in the length of REM stages after 0.5 mg brotizolam and in the wash-out night after 0.5 mg brotizolam reached also the level of statistical significance as compared with placebo as well as with the wash-out night after placebo administration (fig. 4).

Movement time exhibited a trend towards a reduction after placebo, 0.2 and 0.5 mg brotizolam and 30 mg flurazepam, but the findings did not reach the level of statistical significance.

Sleep latency (= time until the appearance of the first 3 consecutive 30-s epochs with stage 2) was shortened in all recorded drug nights and wash-out nights as compared with the baseline which reached the level of statistical significance after 0.5 mg brotizolam as well as in the wash-out nights after 0.1, 0.2 and 0.5 mg brotizolam and 30 mg flurazepam. However, the decrease in sleep latency after 0.1 and 0.2 mg brotizolam was significantly less than after placebo.

The number of *nightly awakenings* ('middle insomnia') demonstrated a dose-dependent, significant decrease after brotizolam as well as after 30 mg flurazepam, while no changes occurred after placebo as compared with baseline (fig. 5). The drug-induced decrease in the number of awakenings reached also the level of statistical significance as compared with placebo.

2. Subjective Sleep Variables

Sleep comfort demonstrated a dose-dependent improvement after brotizolam as well as after flurazepam, with the latter reaching the level of statistical significance ($p < 0.05$, Wilcoxon test) (table I).

Deep sleep was felt to be significantly augmented after 0.2 and 0.5 mg brotizolam which reached the level of statistical significance as compared with the baseline as well as with the placebo nights (table I). *Light sleep,* on the other hand, was significantly reduced by 0.2 and 0.5 mg brotizolam as well as by mg flurazepam, which reached the level of statistical significance as compared with placebo after 0.2 mg brotizolam and 30 mg flurazepam. *Early insomnia* (difficulties in falling asleep) decreased significantly after all active compounds as compared with the baseline. *Restlessness* during the night was reduced by 0.2 mg brotizolam as compared with baseline and placebo. *Middle insomnia* was decreased in the wash-out night following 30 mg flurazepam as compared with the placebo wash-out night. *Difficulties in getting back to sleep* after nightly awakenings were reduced after 0.2 and 0.5 mg brotizolam and after 30 mg flurazepam as well as in the wash-out after 30 mg flurazepam as compared with placebo and the placebo wash-out night, respectively. *Sleep latency* as estimated by the subjects themselves in minutes was reduced by 0.2 and 0.5 mg brotizolam and 30 mg flurazepam with the changes reaching the level of statistical significance as compared with placebo after 0.5 mg brotizolam and 30 mg flurazepam.

Table I. Changes in the subjectively evaluated quality of awakening in the morning after single doses of WE 941, 30 mg flurazepam, and placebo. Increase or decrease at $p < 0.05$ as compared with as compared with ± baseline, (±) placebo, [±] placebo-withdrawal

	0.1 mg		0.2 mg		0.5 mg		Flurazepam	
	night 2	night 3	night 4	night 5	night 6	night 7	night 8	night 9
Comfortable sleep?							+	
Deep sleep?			+		+			
			(+)		(+)			
Light sleep?			–		–		–	
			(–)				(–)	
Insomnia early?	–		–		–		–	
Restlessness during			–					
night?			(–)					
Insomnia middle?								[–]
Difficulty getting back to sleep?			(–)		(–)		(–)	[–]
Pleasant dreams?								
Bad dreams?								
Estimated sleep latency,			–		–		–	
min					(–)		(–)	
Number of awakenings			–		–		–	
			(–)		(–)		(–)	
Number of dream periods							–	
Total length of dreams							–	
Wakefulness before		[–]	–		–		–	
waking signal			(–)		(–)		(–)	

The *number of awakenings* decreased significantly after 0.2 and 0.5 mg brotizolam and 30 mg flurazepam as compared with both placebo and the baseline night. The *number of dream periods* was reduced significantly by 30 mg flurazepam as compared with placebo as was the *total length of dreams. Wakefulness before the waking signal* was reduced by 0.2 and 0.5 mg brotizolam and 30 mg flurazepam as compred with placebo and the baseline night, but was also reduced in the wash-out night after 0.1 mg brotizolam as compared with the placebo wash-out night (table I).

3. Subjective Quality of Awakening in the Mornings (Sleep Questionnaire)

The subjectively experienced quality of awakening in the morning was not altered significantly by any of the substances as compared with baseline. The only significant change was a decrease in good mood after 0.1 mg brotizolam as compared with placebo.

4. Objective Quality of Awakening in the Morning (Psychometry)

Psychometric variables exhibited generally only a few statistically significant changes as compared with the baseline morning as well as with the morning after placebo administration.

Attention (as evaluated based on the total score in the AD test) was improved after all adminstered substances as compared with baseline, which reached the level of statistical significance only in the wash-out night after 0.2 mg brotizolam. *Concentration and attention variability* did not change significantly. *Psychomotor activity* (as evaluated based on the psychomotor activity test of *Grünberger* [1977] demonstrated in the right hand after 0.2 mg brotizolam and 30 mg flurazepam a decrease as compared with the baseline night but not as compared with the placebo night ($p < 0.05$ and 0.01, respectively, t-test). In the left hand a reduction in psychomotor activity was seen after 0.5 mg brotizolam, but again this was not significant as compared with placebo. *CFF* did not show any significant changes. *Reaction time* (in ms) was significantly lengthened after 0.2 mg brotizolam as compared with baseline and placebo. As in the other psychometric variables, there were not significant findings in the Newman-Keuls test. The *reaction time quotient* remained unchanged. *Mood* (as evaluated by the von Zerssen scale) demonstrated no significant changes.

5. Dose-Efficacy Relations

In order to evaluate the predictive potential of the quantitative pharmaco-EEG method in early clinical drug evaluations of hypnotics, we compared the dose-efficacy relations based on 9 wake EEG variables (delta, $theta_1$, $theta_2$, $alpha_1$, $alpha_2$, $beta_1$, $beta_2$, $beta_3$ and $beta_4$) with those based on 9 objective sleep variables (stages W, 1, 2, 3, 4, REM, MT, sleep latency and number of awakenings) and 9 subjective sleep variables (comfortable sleep, deep sleep, light sleep, sleep latency, number of awakenings, diffuculty in getting back to sleep, number of dreams, total length of dreams, awakefulness before wakening signal) (fig. 6). Further dose-efficacy relations were calculated based on changes in 9 objective and 9 subjective variables regarding the quality of awakening in the morning (fig. 7). These relations were calculated by means of a Friedman's rank Anova and multiple Wilcoxon test based on sign-free changes from the baseline in the above-mentioned variables.

As seen in figure 6, the dose-efficacy relations based on wake-EEG variables are indeed similar to the ones established by means of objective and subjective sleep variables. In all 3 instances, 0.5 mg brotizolam is more efficient than 0.2 (or 0.3) mg which in turn is more effective than 0.1 mg. 0.5 mg brotizolam differs significantly from placebo but also from 0.1 and 0.3 mg but not from 30 mg flurazepam based on *all* wake and *all* sleep EEG variables.

Based on subjective sleep variables, both 0.5 mg brotizolam and 30 mg flurazepam differ from placebo and 0.1 mg brotizolam. Thus, the dose-efficacy rela-

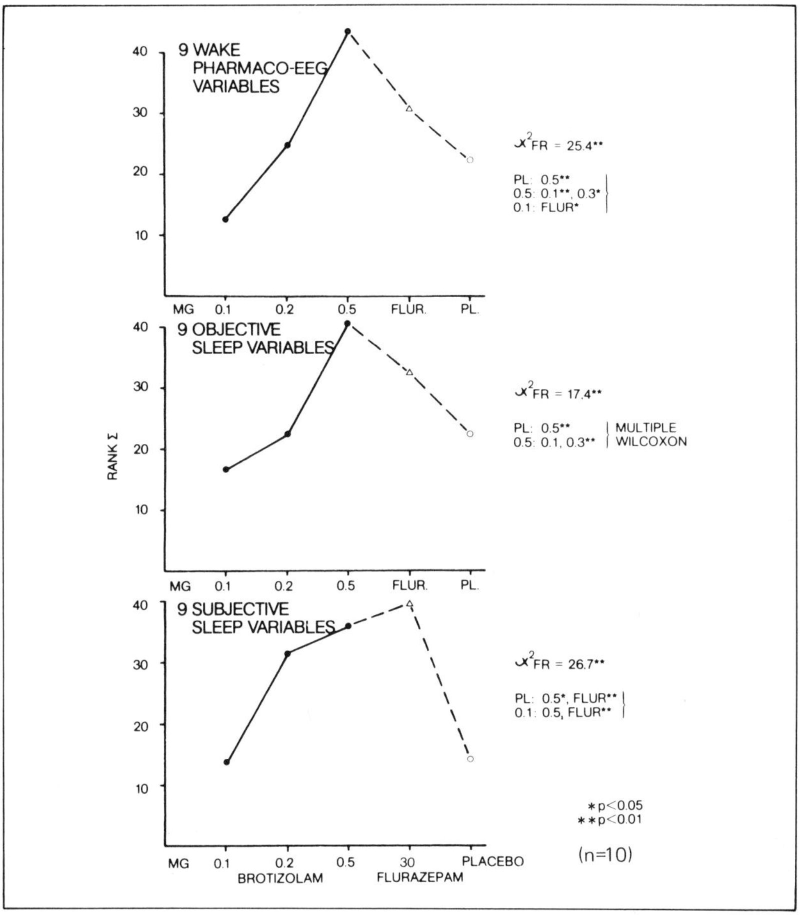

Fig. 6. Dose-efficacy relations of brotizolam (based on Friedman's rank Anova and multiple Wilcoxon test of sign-free changes in either 9 wake pharmaco-EEG variables or 9 objective sleep variables or 9 subjective sleep variables). Drugs are represented in the abscissa, encephaloptropic and psychotropic effects are shown in terms or rank sums in the ordinates. Note the similarity in the different dose-efficacy relations. Only 0.5 mg brotizolam can be differentiated from placebo by *all* 3 evaluation techniques.

tions based on wake EEG data were confirmed by our all-night sleep investigations.

Dose-efficacy relations regarding quality of awakening in the morning were determined based on sign-free changes in 9 subjective variables (difficulty in getting alert; refreshed; ecxhausted; good mood; bad mood; nausea; headaches;

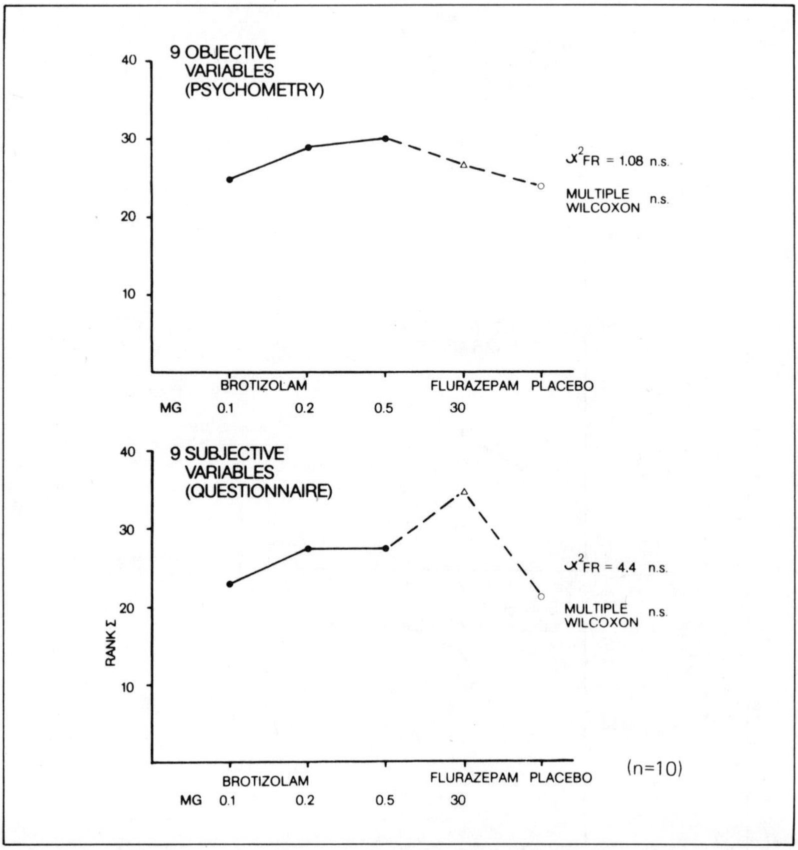

Fig. 7. Dose-efficacy relations regarding the quality of awakening in the morning after brotizolam based on 9 objective variables (psychometry) and 9 subjective variables (questionnaire). Doses are shown in the abscissa, drug-induced changes are seen in terms of rank sums in the ordinates. There are no significant differences between the substances suggesting good tolerance of brotizolam and flurazepam.

dryness of mouth; dizziness; ataxia) and in 9 objective (psychometric) variables (attention, concentration, attention variability, psychomotor activity – right hand ; psychomotor activity – left hand; reaction time – ms; reaction time quotient; flicker frequency – descending value and mood based on the von Zerssen rating scale). There were no significant differences between the drugs and placebo nor between the druggs themselves (fig. 7). Thus, all substances were well tolerated.

6. Correlations between Objective and Subjective Sleep and Awakening Variables

Correlating objective and subjective variables we observed that sleep comfort was negatively correlated with stage REM, 1, 4, movement time and number of nightly awakenings, while positively correlated with stage 2 (table II); e.g. the more stage 2 a subject had in his all-night sleep record, the better rested he felt on the next morning. Furthermore, the more stage 2 and the less stage REM, stage 1 and MT in the sleep polygram, the deeper the subject felt that he slept. In contrast, 'light' sleep was negatively correlated with stages 1, 4, W and sleep latency and negatively with stage 2. The less stage 3 and the more stage W and number of nocturnal awakenings in the sleep record, the more restlessness the subject rated himself. Difficulties to sleep throughout the night (middle insomnia) were negatively correlated with stage 2 and 3 and positively so with stage W and number of nocturnal awakenings. Difficulties to get back to sleep after nightly awakenings were correlated with the feelings of exhaustion on the next morning. Further relations between subjective and objective sleep variables are given in table II.

Discussion

Our all-night polygraphical investigations demonstrated that brotizolam (WE 941) produced significant changes in the sleep profile as compared with the baseline night, which were characterized by a dose-dependent decrease in stages W (intermittent wakefulness), 1, REM, and number of nightly awakenings as well as by an increase in stage 2. Similar changes were induced also by the reference hypnotic drug 30 mg flurazepam which confirms our own [*Saletu,* 1976] and other's investigations [*Kales* et al., 1969, 1970a, b]. Thus, our findings are generally in accordance with the literature on the changes of the sleep profile by anxiolytic sedatives [*Saletu,* 1976].

There were no rebound effects in the wash-out night after brotizolam as compared with placebo, while in the wash-out night after 30 mg flurazepam similar alterations were observed as in the drug-night itself (decrease of stage 1, increase of stage 2), which suggests once again a long-lasting CNS effect of flurazepam due to its long half-life of its active metabolite *N*-desalkylflurazepam [*Breimer,* 1979].

Dose-efficacy relations based on *all* objective sleep variables demonstrated that 0.2 mg brotizolam produced only slighty more effects than 0.1 mg, while 0.5 mg was double as effective as 0.2 mg. However, only 0.5 mg was significantly different from placebo, as there were significant differences between the two low doses and the higher one. On the other hand, no difference could be observed at a level of statistical significance between 0.5 mg brotizolam and 30 mg

Table II. Significant correlation between objective and subjective sleep parameters

	S1 REM	S2 St1	S3 St2	S4 St3	S5 St4	S6 MT	S7 W	S8 SL	S9 NoW
Comfortable sleep?	– *	– ***	+ **		– **	– *			– **
Deep sleep?	– **	– **	+ **			– *			
Light sleep?			– *				+ **		+ *
Insomnia early?		+ **	– ***		+ *		+ ***	+ ***	
Restlessness during night?			–	– *			+ **		+ **
Insomnia middle?			– *	– *			+ ***		+ ***
Difficulty getting back to sleep?	– *	+ *					+ ***		+ ***
Pleasant dreams?							+ ***	+ *	
Bad dreams?			– **		+ *	– **	+ **	+ ***	
Refreshed?			+ *						
Exhausted?				+ *	+ *			+ *	– *

* $p \leqslant 0.05$; ** $p \leqslant 0.01$; *** $p \leqslant 0.001$.

flurazepam. Our dose-efficacy relations strikingly resemble those already described much earlier based on quantitative pharmaco-EEG investigations in wake, normal subjects [*Saletu* et al., 1979]. In the latter pharmaco-EEG investigations we predicted that: (1) WE 941 is significantly CNS effective as compared with placebo; (2) that its pharmaco-EEG profile is that of an anxiolytic sedative, and (3) that the dosage of 0.5 mg and eventually of 0.3 mg should be clinically tried in sleep studies, while 0.1 mg brotizolam should be investigated as tranquilizing medication.

Indeed, the dose-efficacy relations based on drug-induced changes in wake pharmaco-EEG and all-night variables are almost identical even in regard to the equipotency of brotizolam to flurazepam. While the latter positioned itself in

Table II. (continued)

	S1 REM	S2 St1	S3 St2	S4 St3	S5 St4	S6 MT	S7 W	S8 SL	S9 NoW
Good mood?					– *		+ *		
Bad mood?			– *		+ *	– **	+ *	+ ***	– **
Headaches?			+ *				– *	– *	
Dryness of mouth?	+ ***	– *							– **
Dizziness?	– *								– **
Movements uncoordinated					+ *			+ **	– **
Estimated sleep latency			– *			+ **	+ ***	+ ***	
Number of awakenings	+ *				– *				+ ***
Number of dream periods		+ *	– *		– *				
Total length of dreams		+ **	– *		– *				

* $p \leq 0.05$; ** $p \leq 0.01$; *** $p \leq 0.001$.

both studies between the high (0.5 mg) and the middle (0.3 and 0.2 mg) dosage of brotizolam, 0.5 mg brotizolam differed from all the administered substances but 30 mg brotizolam. Our findings indicate that the quantitative pharmaco-EEG is a good predictor in early clinical drug evaluation of hypnotic substances.

Evaluation of the subjective sleep variables revealed that the sleep quality was improved by brotizolam administered in doses between 0.2 and 0.5 mg as well as by 30 mg flurazepam, while 0.1 mg brotizolam did not exert any significant effect as compared with placebo. These variables were characterized by the subjects' reports about more deep sleep, less light sleep, less initial, middle and late insomnia, less difficulty to get back to sleep after night awakenings.

After awakening in the morning, the subjects felt no hangover after any of the substances as compared with placebo, which was documented by a lack of subjective complaints as well as of significant alterations in psychometric variables such as attention, concentration, attention variability, psychomotor activity (right and left hand), reaction time, reaction time quotient, CFF and mood. Further evidence for a good tolerance of brotizolam lies in the fact that the active drugs could not be differentiated from placebo based on subjective and objective sleep variables in the morning. This confirms again our quantitative pharmaco-EEG results in the wake state, as the augmentation of slow activity (= sedative effect) lasted 6–8 h.

Finally, we collected further evidence that drug-induced changes in objective sleep variables are correlated to such in subjective sleep variables. Specifically, we found sleep comfort negatively correlated with stage REM, 1, 4, MT and number of awakenings, while positively correlated with stage 2. The more stage 2 and the less stages REM, 1 and MT, the 'deeper' the sleep as rated by the subjects themselves. On the other hand, 'light' sleep was negatively correlated with stage 2 and positively so with stage W and number of awakenings. Difficulties to sleep through the night were positively correlated with stages W and number of awakenings and negatively so with stages 2 and 3. The feeling of being refreshed in the morning was positively correlated with stage 2. Our findings confirm our own previous results [*Saletu,* 1975] as well as those of *Lienert and Othmer* [1965] that subjects feeling refreshed in the morning had remained significantly longer in a medium depth of sleep (stage 2) than nonrefreshed sleepers.

Summary

Based on quantitative pharmaco-EEG and psychometric studies involving brotizolam (WE 941) – a new triazolothienodiazepine – we had predicted that: (1) the drug is CNS-effective in doses of 0.1–0.5 mg; (2) it is an anxiolytic sedative; (3) 0.1 mg may be regarded as a tranquilizing dose, while 0.3 but especially 0.5 mg exert an additional sleep-inducing effect; (4) the sedative effect lasts 6–8 h, as slow activity was significantly augmented up to this time.

In a subsequent double-blind, placebo-controlled, all-night sleep EEG investigation these predictions were put to the test. 10 normal healthy volunteers spent 13 nights in the laboratory: 2 adaptation nights, 1 baseline night, 5 drug nights (0.1, 0.2, 0.5 mg WE 941, 30 mg flurazepam and placebo) and 5 wash-out nights. Drugs were administered in 3-day intervals in a randomized fashion. Objective sleep variables were recorded between 10.30 p.m. and 6 a.m. and were evaluated according to the criteria of *Rechtschaffen and Kales.* Subjective quality of sleep and of the morning awakening was rated by means of a questionnaire, while the objective quality of morning awakening was assessed by means of a psychometric test battery. WE 941 induced a decrease in stages W, 1 and REM, as well as an increase in stages 2 which reached the level of statistical significance as compared with placebo only after the highest dose. The number of awakenings were significantly and dose-dependently reduced. 30 mg flurazepam produced similar alterations which – quite in contrast to WE 941 – could partially still be observed in the wash-out nights (long half-life!). Subjective sleep quality was not changed by 0.1 mg WE 941, while it was found to be improved after 0.2 and 0.5 mg WE 941 and 30 mg flurazepam. Dose-efficacy relations based on *all* sleep variables strikingly resembled those obtained in the wake state, suggesting that the quantitative pharmaco-EEG method is of predictive value in early clinical evaluation of hypnotic drugs. The subjective quality of awakening in the morning remained unchanged as compared with the baseline and placebo nights (no 'hangover'), which was confirmed by psychometric tests including the evaluation of attention, concentration, attention variability, psychomotor activity, CFF, reaction time and mood. Finally correlations between objective and subjective sleep and awakening variables were investigated.

Acknowledgement

The authors would like to express their thanks to Dr. *von Delbrück,* MD, of C.H. Boehringer Sohn; to Dr. *R. Flener,* MD, and Ms. *A. Kalk* of Bender and Co.; to Dr. *L. Linzmayer,* PhD, to *Ruth Wolff,* Secretary, and to the entire staff of the Section of Pharmacopsychiatry and of the Sleep Laboratory at the Psychiatrische Universitätsklinik Wien for their valuable assistance.

References

Boehringer, Ingelheim: WE 941 – zentrales Depressivum. Investigational Brochure (1976).

Breimer, D.D.: Clinical pharmacokinetic and biopharmaceutical aspects of hypnotic drug therapy; in Priest, Pletscher, Ward, Sleep research, pp. 63–81 (MTP Press, Lancaster 1979).

Fink, M.: EEG and human psychopharmacology. A. Rev. Pharmacol. *9:* 241–258 (1969).

Grünberger, J.: Psychodiagnostik des Alkoholkranken. Methodischer Beitrag zur Bestimmung der Organizität in der Psychiatrie (Maudrich, Wien 1977).

Grünberger, J.; Saletu, B.; Linzmayer, L.; Kalk, A.; Berner, P.: Pharmacodynamic investigations with WE 941, a new triazolodiazepine, by means of psychometric analyses. Curr. ther. Res. *24:* 427–440 (1978).

Herrmann, W.M.; Fichte, K.; Itil, T.M.; Kubicki, S.: Acute efficacy of 20 psychotropic drugs on human EEG power spectrum variables shown by multivariate and univariate statistics; in Saletu, Berner, Hollister, Neuro-psychopharmacology, pp. 371–381 (Pergamon Press, Oxford 1979).

Itil, T.M.: Quantitative pharmco-electroencephalography. Mod. Probl. Pharmacopsychiat., vol. 8, pp. 43–75 (Karger, Basel 1974).

Kales, A.; Allen, C.; Scharf, M.B.; Kales, J.D.: Hypnotic drugs and their effectiveness. All-night EEG studies of insomniac subjects. Archs gen. Psychiat. *23:* 226–232 (1970a).

Kales, A.; Kales, J.D.; Scharf, M.B.; Tan, T.L.: Hypnotics and altered sleep-dream patterns. II. All-night EEG studies of chloral hydrate, flurazepam, and methaqualone. Archs gen. Psychiat. *23:* 219–225 (1970b).

Kales, A.; Malmstrom, E.J.; Kee, H.K.; Kales, J.D.; Tan, T.L.: Effects of hypnotics on sleep patterns, dreaming and mood state: labaratory and home studies. Biol. Psychiat. *1:* 235–241 (1969).

Lienert, G.A.; Othmer, E.: Objective correlates of the refreshing effects of sleep. Prog. Brain Res. *18:* 170–174 (1965).

Osgood, C.D.; Suci, G.J.; Tannenbaum, P.H.: The measurement of meaning (University Press, Urbana 1975).

Rechtschaffen, A.; Kales, A.: A manual of standardized terminology, techniques and scoring system for sleep stages of human subjects. Publ. No. 204 (National Institute of Health, Bethesda 1968).

Saletu, B.: Is the subjectively experienced quality of sleep related to objective sleep parameters? Behav. Biol. *13:* 433–444 (1975).

Saletu, B.: Psychopharmaka, Gehirntätigkeit und Schlaf (Karger, Basel 1976).

Saletu, B.: Quantitatives Pharmako-EEG. Eine Methode zur Klassifikation und Bestimmung der Pharmakodynamik von Psychopharmaka; in Langer, Berner, Psychopharmakologisches Seminar 1978/79 der Psychiatrischen Universitätsklinik Wien (Maudrich, Wien 1981).

Saletu, B.; Allen, M.; Itil, T.M.: The effect of coca-cola, daffeine, antidepressants and chlorpromazine on objective and subjective sleep paramenters. Pharmakopsychiatr. Neuro-Psychopharmakol. *7:* 307–321 (1974).

Saletu, B.; Grünberger, J.; Volavka, J.; Berner, P.: Classification and bioavailability studies with WE 941 by quantitative pharmaco-EEG and clinical analysis. Arzneimittel-Forsch. *29:* 700–704 (1979).

Saletu, B.; Matjecek, M.; Knor, K.; Ferner, U.; Schneewind, U.: Assessing the psychoactiving of cloxazolam (MT-14411) by quantitative EEG and psychological studies. Curr. ther. Res. *20:* 510–528 (1976).

Saletu, B.; Taeuber K.: Serum levels of nomifensine and pharmacodynamics assessed by the computer-pharmaco-EEG; in Stonier, Jenner, Nomifensine, pp. 31–38 (Academic Press/ Royal Society of Medicine, London 1980).

Weber, K.H.; Bauer, A.; Langbein, A.; Daniel, H.: Heteroaromaten mit anellierten Siebenringen. III. Umwandlung von Thienotriazolooxazepinen in Diazepine. Liebigs Annln Chem. pp. 1257–1265 (1978).

Zerssen, V.D. von: Koeller, D.M.; Rey, E.R.: Die Befindlichkeitsskala (B-S) – ein einfaches Instrument zur Objektivierung von Befindlichkeitsstörungen, insbesondere im Rahmen von Längsschnittuntersuchungen, Arzneimittel-Forsch. *20:* 915–918 (1970).

Univ. Doz. Dr. Bernd Saletu, Head, Section of Pharmacopsychiatry,
Psychiatrische Universitätsklinik Vienna, Währingergürtel 74–76,
A-1090 Vienna (Austria)

Adv. biol. Psychiat., vol. 6, pp. 143–153 (Karger, Basel 1981)

Some Aspects on Geometrical Spectral Descriptors of the EEG[1]

J. Cumberbatch, L. von Knorring, C. Perris[2]
Umeå Data Center, University of Umeå, Department of Psychiatry,
University of Umeå, Umeå, Sweden

Introduction

The data registered during an EEG recording is of such volume that unless a data reduction is performed it is impractical to attempt an analysis, even with the aid of a computer. Presented here are some aspects on how to effectively reduce the data volume yet at the same time retain the information content of the original signals.

Method

In EEG analysis of the type discussed here, six electrodes, denoted channels 1 through 6 (F3, F4, C3, C4, 01, and 02 according to the international 10–20 system), have been used. After amplification the signals derived are plotted on paper and are also recorded on magnetic tape. A visual examination of the plotted signals enables possible distortion, such as electrode and muscle artifacts, to be detected. The signals are then digitalized with the exclusion of all distortion. As an aid to data reduction the Fourier transform is used. The application of the Fourier Transform to EEG analysis has been discussed by many authors (for instance Etevenon (1978) and Walter (1963)). Only a few aspects will be discussed here. The Fourier Transform is a mathematical operation which converts a time dependent founction into a frequency dependent function. The number of calculation which must be performed can be greatly reduced if the Fast Fourier Transform (FFT) is used.

As an example of the FFT consider the wave form shown in figure 1. The wave form is that of a sine wave having a frequency of 6 Hz. By digitalizing a 4-s segment of the sine wave (using a sampling frequency of 133 Hz) the FFT reveals the frequency spectrum shown in figure 2. The dominant frequency component is at 6 Hz, corresponding to the original sine wave frequency.

[1] Supported in part by grants from the Swedish Medical Research Council, Grants No. 2568 and 5740.

[2] The skilful technical assistance of Mrs. *Sonja Holmgren* is gratefully acknowledged.

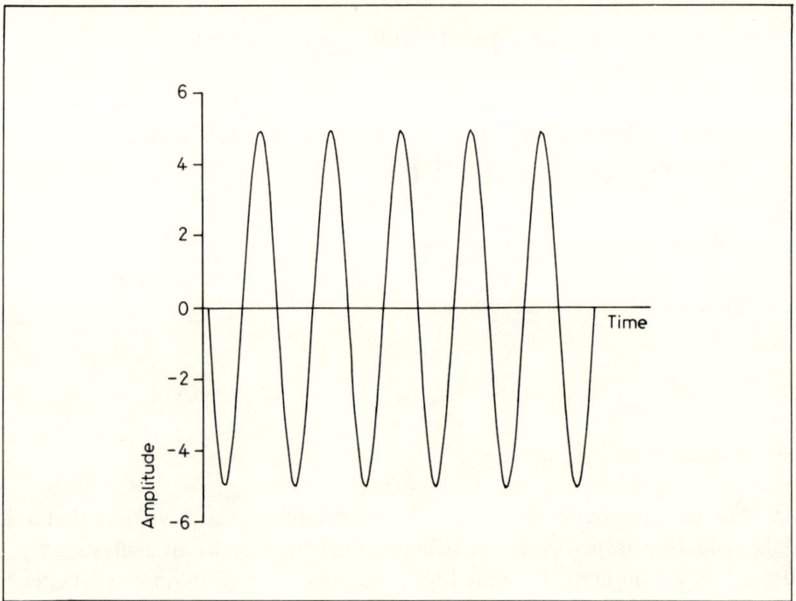

1

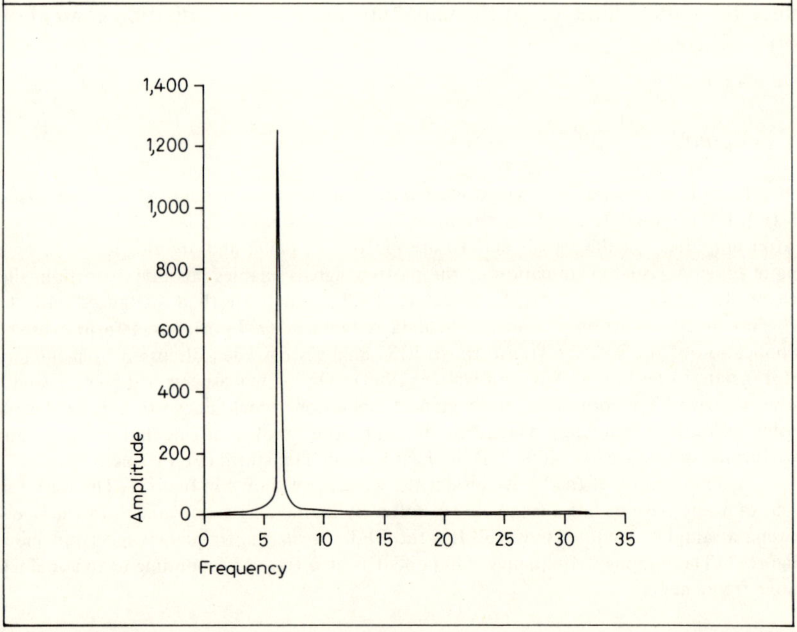

2

Fig. 1. A sine wave having a frequency of 6 Hz.
Fig. 2. The frequency spectrum of the sine wave shown in figure 1.

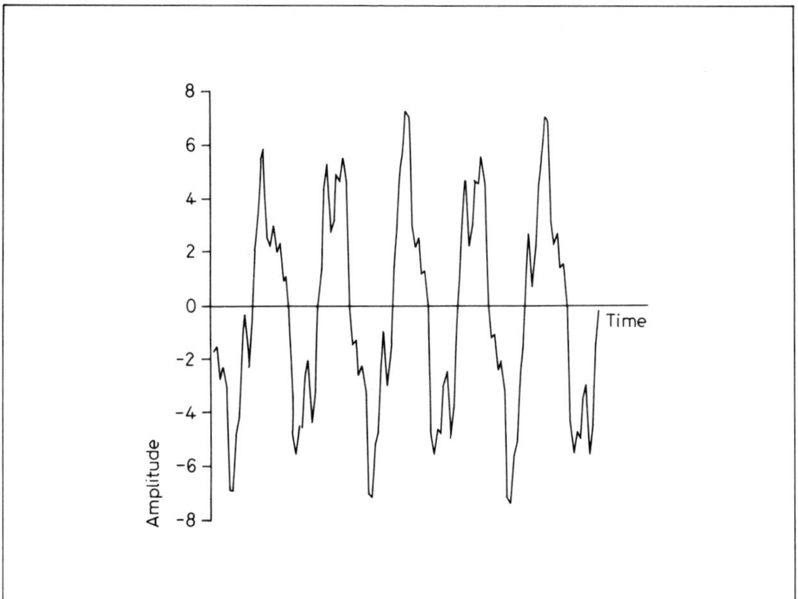

3

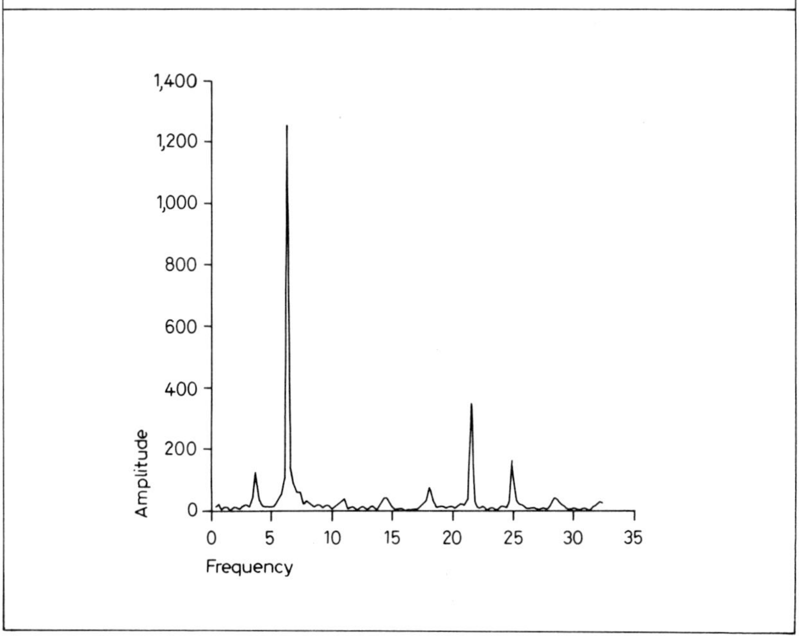

4

Fig. 3. A sine wave, having a frequency of 6 Hz, with uncorrelated noise added. The noise has an amplitude equal to half that of the sine wave.

Fig. 4. The frequency spectrum of the distorted sine wave shown in figure 3.

During the recording of EEG signals every attempt is made to minimize distortion. Yet what if distortion is present? In figure 3 the same sine wave is shown, as in figure 1, but with random distortion added. The distortion represents uncorrelated noise with an amplitude equal to half that of the sine wave. Using the same techniques as before the FFT reveals the frequency spectrum shown in figure 4. The 6 Hz peak is still dominant, although other frequency components are now present. It is important to observe that the aformentioned other frequency components have nothing to do with the 6Hz sinewave. When frequency spectra are calculated caution must be exercised in the interpretation of the results. Some frequency components may be simply the result of the presence of noise.

Spectral Descriptors

Once the frequency spectrum is obtained a set of spectral descriptors can be calculated. The descriptors proposed by *Marciano and Nolfe* [1977] bring about a high degree of data reduction. They convey information about the relative activity (relative mean power), the barycentric frequency (weighted mean frequency) and the barycentric radius (mean band width). Although the descriptors have been used in several applications [*Kemali* et al., 1980] they would not appear to be complete.

All the wave forms shown in figure 5 have the same descriptor values. Yet a visual examination reveals that the wave forms differ in, not least, the number of frequency components (peaks). (Additionally figures 5c and 5d are not symmetrical about the barycentric frequency.) It is therefore suggested that the descriptors proposed by *Marciano and Nolfe* [1977] be complemented with a count of the frequency components in the spectrum. The logic of such, as applied to the analysis presented here, has been to count all deviations of 20% or more of the total amplitude deviation as frequency components. (The figure of 20% is, of course, open to discussion.)

For practical purposes the EEG signals, as discussed here, have been digitalized using a sampling frequency of 133 Hz and then divided up into a number of so-calles epochs each of 3.8 s duration. The FFT is then applied to each epoch and the resulting frequency spectra averaged over all epochs. Additionally the frequency spectrum has been divided into four bands (delta, 1–3.9 Hz; theta, 4.1–7.5 Hz; alpha, 7.5–13.25 Hz, and beta, 13.25–32 Hz). One such frequency spectrum, for channel 1, is shown in figure 6, together with the corresponding values of the spectral descriptors.

One of the problems experienced with counting frequency components is exemplified in figure 6. There is a component exactly on the theta-alpha boundary. Currently such components are not counted. Further research is needed, but it may be appropriate to count such components as belonging to the band in which their maximum value occurs.

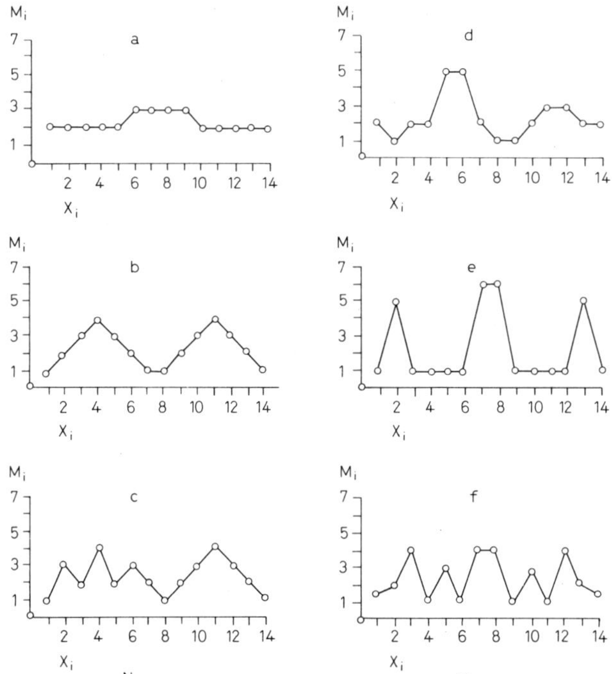

Activity: $\bar{m} = \frac{1}{N}\sum_{i=1}^{N} m_i$ Barycentric frequency: $\bar{x} = \frac{1}{Nm}\sum_{i=1}^{N} m_i x_i$

Barycentric radius: $k = \left[\frac{1}{Nm}\sum_{i=1}^{N} (x_i - \bar{x})^2 m_i\right]^{1/2}$

Fig. 5. In all the above figures (n = 14) the spectral descriptors $\bar{m}$, $\bar{x}$ and k have the same values (2.3, 7.5 and 3.8 respectively). Yet the figures differ in at least two ways: (1) the number of peaks (varies from 1 to 5); (2) symmetry about the barycentric frequency (c and d are not symmetrical).

Stability

If the spectral descriptors are to be representative of the subject undergoing EEG analysis then the frequency spectrum upon which they are calculated must be stable. An investigation has been made of the number of epochs (each of 3.8 s duration) needed to obtain stable frequency spectra. If the EEG curve is regarded as being stable then it is clear from a mathematical point of view that the greater is the number of epochs the more stable are the resulting frequency spectra and the ideal number of epochs needed may be calculated (Jenkins and Watts, –68).

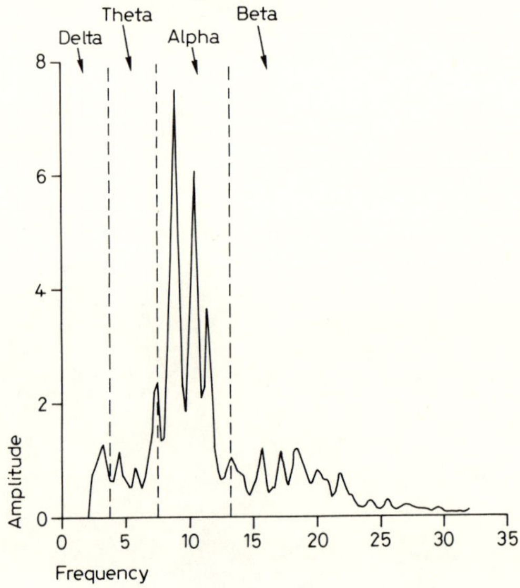

	Delta	Theta	Alpha	Beta
Activity	0.06	0.12	0.55	0.27
Frequency	3.02	6.12	10.02	19.42
Radius	0.45	1.18	1.31	4.17
Components	1.00	1.00	3.00	5.00

Fig. 6. A frequency spectrum (channel 1) averaged over 5 epochs, each of 3.8 s duration, together with corresponding values of spectral descriptors.

However, the EEG curve in a single patient is not stable, changing as a result of changes in vigilance etc. Thus the ideal number of epochs needed to find measures characterising a patient must still be practically investigated in patients.

In the first study two frequency spectra, each averaged over a period of 5 epochs, were calculated for each subject in a group of 7 healthy volunteers. Two such spectra, for one and the same subject (channel 2), are shown in figure 7. A considerable variation in spectral patterns can be seen. Values of the spectral descriptors were then compared for each of the two 5-epoch periods. The percentage difference in the average value of each descriptor over the 7 subjects in the group was then calculated. This percentage difference, for channel 4, is shown in table I. For the 16 descriptors shown in table I, the values differed by on average, 4.4%.

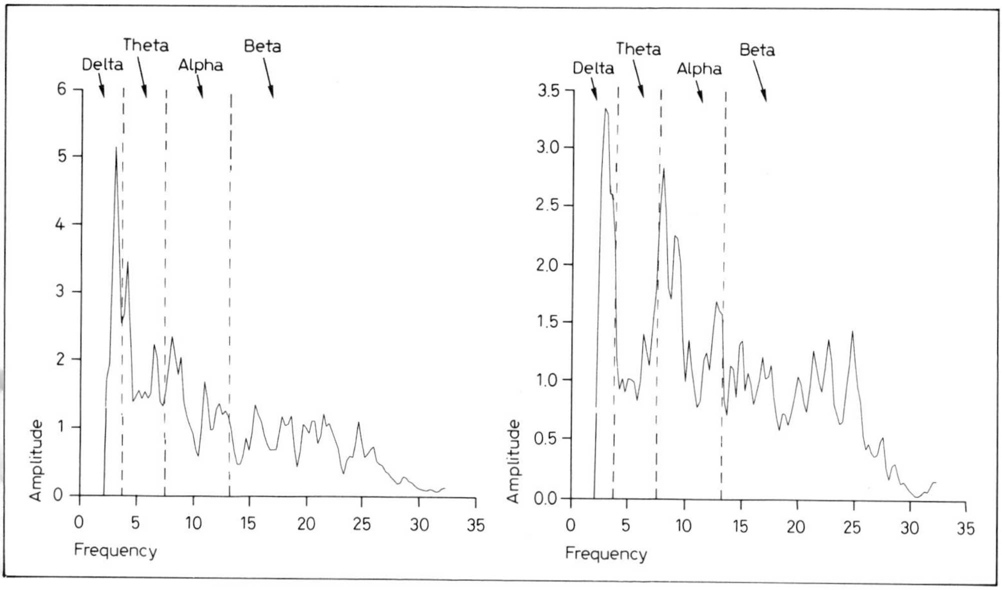

Fig. 7. Frequency spectra (channel 2) averaged over 5 epochs, for one and same subject. Considerable variation in the spectra can be seen, indicating instability.

Table I. Percentage difference in the values of the spectral descriptors averaged over a group of 7 healthy subjects, for two periods of 5 epochs
(channel n = 4)

	Delta %	Theta %	Alpha %	Beta %
Activity	0.0	9.1	0.0	3.6
Frequency	1.4	0.5	0.5	0.5
Radius	8.5	0.0	0.7	1.6
Components	12.3	14.5	8.9	3.6
Average Difference 4.4 %				

In another study of the problem of stability, two frequency spectra, each averaged over a period of 20 epochs, were calculated for each subject in a group of 9 depressed patients. Then for each subject and for each of the two 20-epoch periods the spectral descriptors were calculated. Wilcoxon's matched pair rank sign test was next used to test for significant differences in the respective values

Table II. Percentage differences in the values of the spectral descriptors averaged over a group of 9 depressed subjects, for two periods of 20 epochs (channel n = 4)

	Delta %	Theta %	Alpha %	Beta %
Activity	0.0	4.8	0.0	7.1
Frequency	0.0	0.2	0.2	0.7
Radius	0.0	0.0	0.7	1.3
Components	0.0	14.1	0.0	0.0
Average Difference 1.8 %				

of the spectral descriptors obtained. Only two of the 96 descriptors differed significantly at the 5% level (channel 1, beta, activity and radius). The percentage difference in the average value of each descriptor, over the 9 subjects in the group, was also calculated. The results, for channel 4, are shown in table II. For the 10 descriptors shown in table II the values differed by, on average, 1.8%.

If tables I and II are compared a trend is detected. This trend, together with the results of the Wilcoxon matched pair rank sign test, indicates that after 20 epochs the frequency spectra are becoming stable. *Marciano and Nolfe* [1977] use 40 epochs, and presumably that number is sufficient to ensure that the corresponding spectral descriptors are representative.

Epoch Duration

The question of epoch duration has been partly investigated. For 1 healthy volunteer frequency spectra were calculated, first using 45 epochs, each of 3.8 s duration, and again using 11 epochs, each of 15.2 s duration. The resulting spectra are shown in figure 8, together with the corresponding values of the spectral descpritors. Although the total time duration for the two sepctra is almost the same the number of epochs used, of 15.2 seconds duration, is too few for that spectrum to have stablished. However, this does not detract from the following argument.

Spectra based on epochs of 15.2 s duration are much more detailed than those based on epochs of 3.8 s duration. This is not surprising for such is the property of the FFT. But is the information content of the two spectra shown in figure 8 the same? Might it be that the detailed spectrum is telling us something and that by using epochs of short duration information is lost?

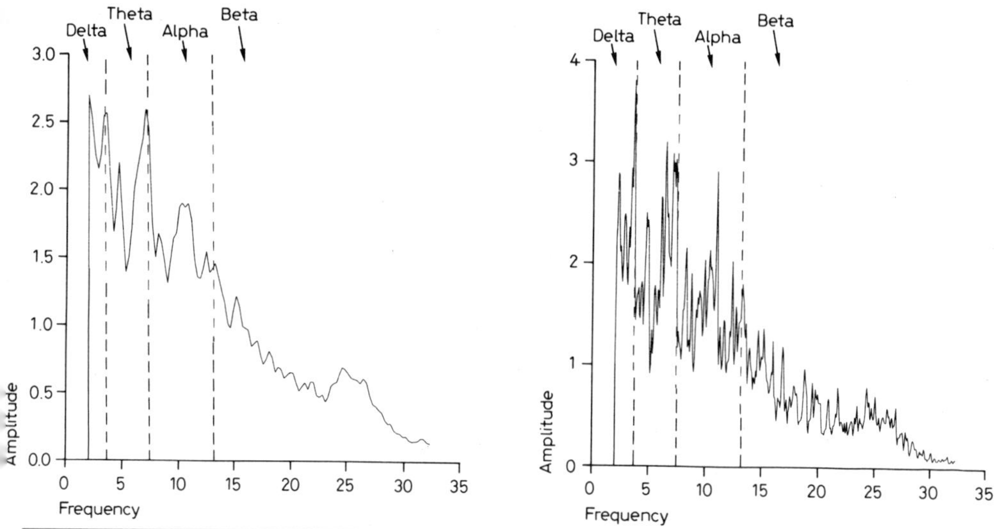

	Delta	Theta	Alpha	Beta
Activity	0.14	0.23	0.29	0.34
Frequency	3.00	5.73	10.07	19.29
Radius	0.52	1.04	1.55	4.64
Components	1.00	1.00	3.00	0.0

	Delta	Theta	Alpha	Beta
Activity	0.15	0.24	0.29	0.33
Frequency	2.91	5.77	10.09	19.33
Radius	0.51	0.95	1.50	4.56
Components	2.00	4.00	9.00	11.00

Fig. 8. On the left is shown a frequency spectrum (channel 2) averaged over 45 epochs, each of 3.8 s duration. On the right is shown a frequency spectrum, for the same subject and channel, averaged over 11 epochs, each of 15.2 s duration. Also shown are the values of the spectral descriptors.

The spectral descriptors, as proposed by *Marciano and Nolfe* [1977], have almost the same values in both spectra. This is a practical example of the problem previously discussed using contructed wave forms. However, the count of the number of frequency components reveals the difference in detail between the two spectra.

Variations within Groups

The spectral descriptions, as discussed here, reduce the data volume to 96 values per subject (16 per channel). Statistical routines are then used to compare values of the spectral descriptors both within and between groups. The results of such comparisons are presented elsewhere [*Perris* et al., 1980].

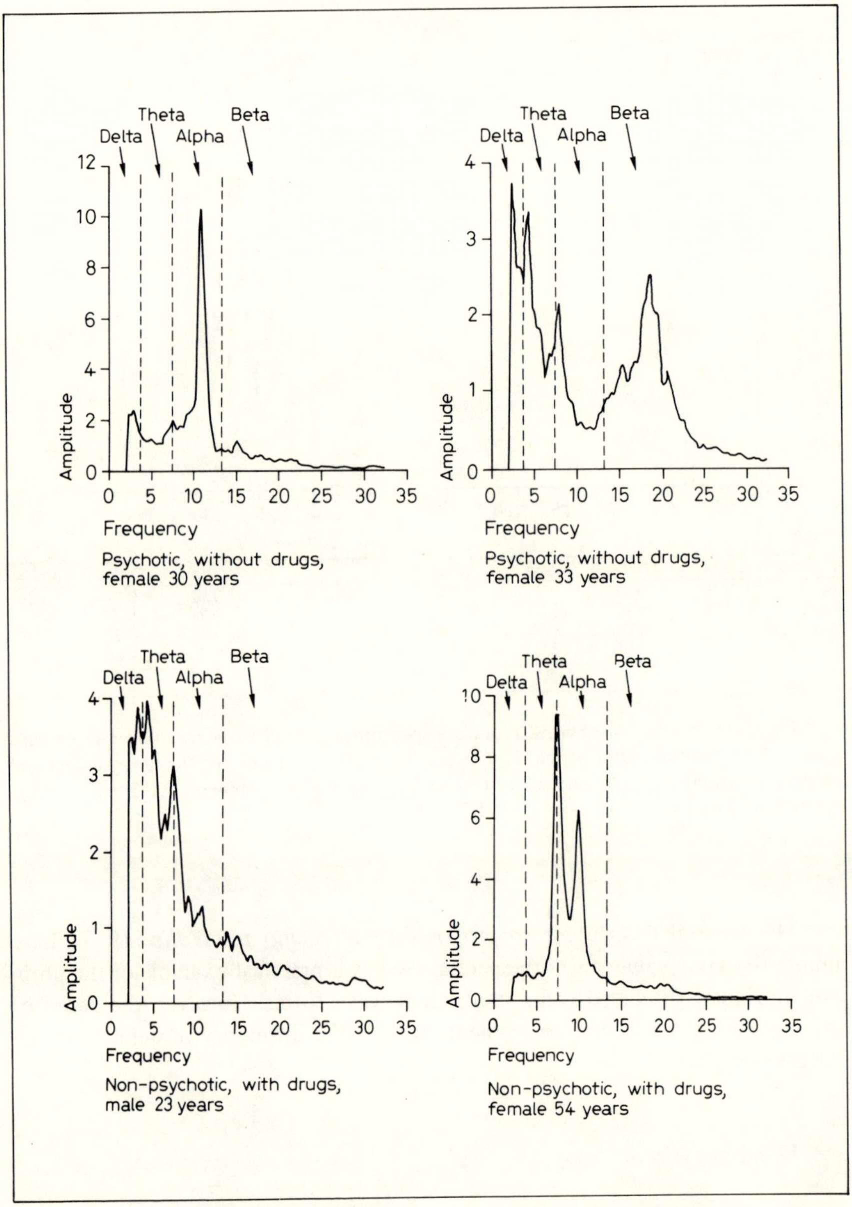

Fig. 9. The frequency spectra (channel 2) for 4 subjects belonging to the same group (depressed). An extreme variation in spectral patterns is seen. Each spectrum is averaged over 20 epochs (3.8 s per epoch).

In figure 9 are shown the frequency spectra, for channel 2, for 4 subjects which, if only broad diagnostic criteria are used, could be classified as belonging to the same group (depressed). Yet an extreme variation in spectral patterns is seen. Even if parameters such as age, sex, diagnostic subgrouping and the presence of drugs are taken into account, large differences in the frequency spectra can still be found. It has, in fact, been previously shown [*Monakhov* et al., 1979] that within such diagnostic categories as psychotic/non-psychotic large differences in symptomatology can exist.

Would it not be appropriate to make the division into subgroups from the homogenity of the frequency spectra found, and then afterwards search for similarities within these groups? The answer to this question, and indeed to many other questions, will come through time and effort. That is research, and it is just as important to be able to raise questions as to be able to answer them.

Summary

The properties of the spectral descriptors, as proposed by Marciano and Nolfe, are examined. It is proposed that the spectral descriptors be complemented with a count of the number of dominant frequency components contained in the EEG signal. The problems of stability and variability in the frequency spectra are discussed.

References

Etevenon, P.: L'electroencephalographie sur ordinateur. Doctoral dissertation, INSERM, Paris 1978.

Jenkins, G., and Watts, D.: Spectral analysis and its applications. Holden-Day (1968).

Kemali, D.; Vacca, L.; Nolfe, G.; Iosio, G.; Carlo, R. de: Hemispheric EEG quantitative asymetrics in schizophrenics and depressed patients. Adv. biol. Psychiat., vol. 4, pp. 14–20 (Karger, Basel 1980).

Marciano, F.; Nolfe, G.: Geometrical spectral descriptors. Internal report No. 7, Institute of Cybernetics, National Council of Research, Naples 1977.

Monakhov, K.; Perris, C.; Botskarev, V.K.; Knorring, L. von; Nikiforov, A.I.: Functional interhemispheric differences in relation to various psychopathological components of the depressive syndromes. A pilot international study. Neuropsychobiology *5:* 143–155 (1979).

Perris, C.; Knorring L. von; Cumberbatch, J.; Marciano, F.: Further studies of depressed patients by means of computerized EEG. Proc. 2nd Symp. on Clinical Neurophysiological Aspects of Psychopathological Conditions, Capri 1980.

Walter, D.O.: Spectral analysis of electroencephalograms: mathematical determination of neurophysiological relationships from records of limited duration. Exp. Neurol. *8:* 155–181, 1963.

C. Perris, MD, Department of Psychiatry, University of Umeå,
S-901 85 Umeå (Sweden)

Adv. biol. Psychiat., vol. 6, pp. 154–164 (Karger, Basel 1981)

Critical Examination on EEG Evoked Potential Utilization

Example of Some Problems Related to the Evaluation of the Auditory Function[1]

M. Bracale[2]

Cattedra di Elettronica Biomedica, Istituto Elettrotecnico, Facoltà di Ingegneria, Napoli, Italia

Introduction

Our brain is connected to the external environment through the sensorial organs which act as transducers, converting physical energy, i.e. existing in the sound or light waves, with a series of pulses transmitted through the nerve fibres to the brain. The intensity or the amplitude of the sensorial stimulus is codified as frequency of the pulses. The acoustic system, for exampie, is roughly shown in figure 1.

The mechanical part is formed by the external, middle and inner ear. While this block is identified enough, there are several points to be clarified about the process concerning the other two blocks.

The functional link between input and output appears through sound sensations. These sensations are generally evaluated subjectively through adequate psyco-physical tests. One of these tests belongs to the determination of the threshold frequency audiogram. Generally, these kind of measurements, even made with enough precision and stability to allow useful interactions with medical physiological observations, still are, sometimes, limited by both subjectivity and several uncertainties. The latter can be caused by several factors directly or indirectly connected to the sensorial function, i.e. training for the test, emotivity, stress, adaptation, background noise, technique measurements, and so on. Therefore, the necessity of alternative or at least complementary techniques that elim-

[1] The present work was supported by National Council of Researches of Rome.

[2] The author wishes to express his appreciation and grateful thanks to Miss *Tiziana Lamanna,* for all assistance in preparing the manuscript.

inate the subjectivity of the evaluations is ever present. This condition becomes necessary when the subject cannot communicate, i.e. (new-born children, mutes, etc.).

In these objective techniques, the measurement aims to determine the answers that represent particular physiological variables related to the auditory function. Particularly, we refer to the modifications affecting EEG when the subject receives short periods and repetitive stimuli. The technique of auditory function evaluation, based on the analysis of acoustic evoked potentials (AEP), is originated by these measurements.

At the moment, there are several commercial systems for determining AEP's but there are many problems involved in such methodologies. In the present paper we want to recall the most important problems emphasizing also that some complications, that are directly connected to the fundamental neurophysiological mechanisms, need further analysis before use with no doubt the confirmation of previous methodology.

Active and Passive Transmission of the Information in the Brain System

The information flow in the brain, as it occurs for other parts of the human being, is mainly due to electrochemical processes that involve cells and neurons with different components, including axons, synapses, dendrites and so on. The transmission of information that occurs in these structures can be named 'active'. The body as a whole, or a particular part of itself, can be considered, from the electrical conductivity point of view, as a conductive mass that can or cannot be isotropic and homogeneous in terms of conductivity. Considering these features and hypothesizing that the brain and its tegumenta are conductive, it is possible to describe the head as a non-homogeneous and, probably, anisotropic volume conductor of finite extension with a self-contained electrical source. The points electrically active produce electric current in the medium or in the surrounding media. If these currents are following in a medium of finite conductivity, they will produce a potential field in the conductive volume. Through an adequate technique of recording it is possible to monitor the resultant potentials. When the two sampling electrodes are located on two disparate isopotential lines, then the potentials generated by these currents represent the transmission of information from the active site to the observer. This is the passive transmission of the information.

The distinction between active and passive transmission must mean that the passive activity does not occur in correspondence of electrically active structures, but somewhere else in the conductive volume. This distinction comes from the field distribution due to generators and to the conductive characteristics of the medium in which the information is propagated.

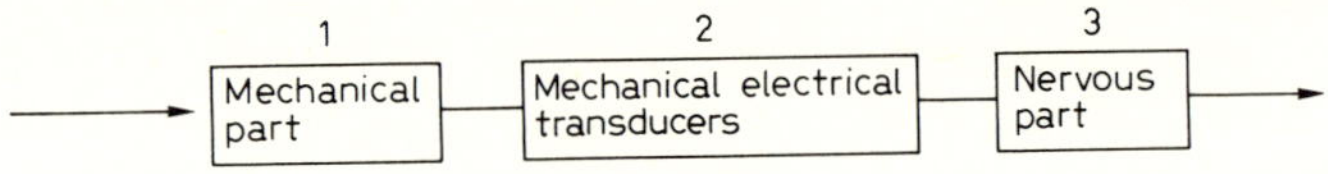

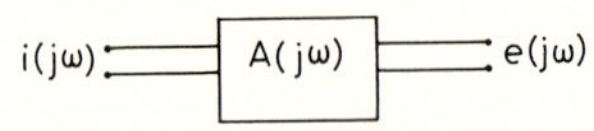

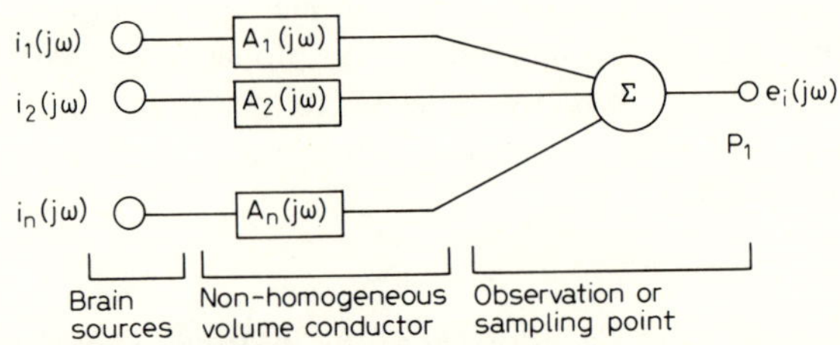

Fig. 1. Schematic block diagram of acoustic system.

Fig. 2. Two-part network representing the non-homogeneous conductive volume of the head.

Fig. 3. An n-dimensional system representing the active sites in the brain and an arbitrary observation point P_1.

The Conduction on the Volume of the Head

If we have only one biogenerator EEG, with particular hypotheses we can consider the output $e(j\omega)$ from a two-part network representing the non-homogeneous conductive volume of the head (fig. 2) wherein $i(j\omega)$ is the input signal in the frequency domain, $e(j\omega)$ is the output signal and $A(j\omega)$ is the 'transfer function'.

According to the hypothesis that the superposition principle is valid for this system, the transfer function of the network operates in a linear fashion on each frequency component of the input signal informing the output signal. Actually we have an n-dimensional system representing the active sites in the brain and an arbitrary observation point P_1 (fig. 3).

For this system, the output signal appearing in P_1 may be written as:

$$e_1(j\omega) = A_1(j\omega)\, i_1(j\omega) + A_2(j\omega)\, i_2(j\omega) + \ldots + A_n(j\omega)\, i_n(j\omega). \quad (1)$$

Since all the sources are distributed in the brain, each fixed in a particular location, the output signal $e_1(j\omega)$ may be termed a spatial superposition of the sources. Each source contributes to the output with a weighting determined by its transfer function.

Of course besides this space superposition, the time superposition is always present due to the fact that the single source can be represented by a series of harmonics:

$$i_i(j\omega) = K_1\, f(j\omega_0) + K_2\, f(2j\omega_0) + \ldots + K_m\, f(mj\omega_0), \tag{2}$$

then:

$$e(j\omega) = \sum_{i=1}^{n} e_i(j\omega) = \sum_{i=1}^{n} A_i(j\omega)\, i_i(j\omega) =$$

$$= \sum_{i=1}^{n} A_i(j\omega)\, |K_1\, f(j\omega_0) + \ldots + K_m\, f(mj\omega_0)|. \tag{3}$$

We have to consider that the n transfer functions are dependent upon a number of variables, i.e. the transfer function $A_K(j\omega)$ is a function both of the K source location, and the picking point, and of the medium inside the non-homogeneous volume conductor. Consequently, we can understand how the problem is considerably complicated in obtaining the identification of the bio-generators that are very numerous in the brain. We can simplify the problem if we limit ourselves, just as a model and in vitro or in vivo measurements, in the identification of only a finite number of sources with known characteristics, taking the information from prefixed points.

It is clear that the limitation is due to the very small number of the possible combinations of picking point sources. Then besides this model approach it seems possible to obtain important information also from direct measurements if we fix, in a standard way, the picking points and if we select in some way the biorhythm sources. It seems that the evoked potential has played a basic role in these measurements. In fact through a proper stimulation over adequate points of peripheral input we can excite defined biogenerators at a central level. Moreover, the averaging technique can eliminate all the remaining activity originated by other generators not correlated with the induced stimulation. Then, through evoked potential analysis we can find, in a principle way, the possibility of selecting the picking points to record an activity originated by well-located generators.

Spontaneous Activity

The human head can be roughly represented as in figure 4, where the different structural layers are shown. It is interesting to note that because the interfaces between the brain and CSF layer, CSF layer and skull, and skull and scalp follow the pattern high-low, low-high and high-low resistance, respectively, that the deviation in outward pathways from what they would be in a homogeneous volume conductor are not as severe as they might be if all the interfaces were of

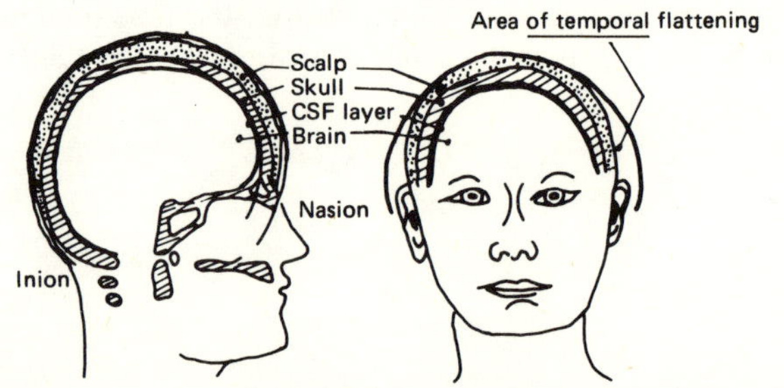

Fig. 4. The structural layers of human head.

the high-low variety. The skull serves to bend currents back toward the radial direction and thereby compensates for the diffractions in the CSF layer and scalp, which are in a direction away from the radial.

From measurements made in vivo and in vitro [*Hoes,* 1970] it has been shown that the closer the source is to the surface, the greater is the radial current and then greater the potential difference in the point.

Imagine a radial line extending from the source through the surface of the scalp. The point where this line intersects the scalp surface represents that point on the scalp that is closest to the source and hence provides a unique reference point. The potential on the scalp due to the radial current component of sources in the brain will be maximized over this reference point and then fall off at points on the scalp away from the reference. The largest potentials at the reference point are obtainable from sources very near the surface of the brain; the amplitudes are reduced for sources more deeply located. Also for sources located near the brain's surface, the potential will fall off much faster away from the reference point than will the potential due to more deeply situated sources. It is this rate at which potential falls off with respect to distance along the scalp surface that determines the magnitude of potential differences that may be measured bipolarly. A bipolar pair will measure a much higher potential difference in the vicinity of the reference point due to a cortical level source than it will due to a thalamic level source. However, due to the rate of potential decrement, the same bipolar pair may measure a potential difference as greater or larger for the thalamic source than for the cortical source at points relatively far-removed (9 cm or farther) from the reference, based upon theoretical predictions.

In addition to effects of source location, it was determined that the non-homogeneous nature of the head provides secondary but not-negligible effects on scalp and cortical potential distributions. Typically, increases in the thickness or resistance of any of the layer surrounding the brain results in reduced scalp potentials, and vice versa.

The major implication for clinical recording practice provided by this work is that the activity measured by electrodes at a specific cortical or scalp location most likely contains or is contaminated with activity due to generators located non-locally with respect to the recording site. When recording a local cortical source with narrowly spaced electrodes it is unlikely that such contamination would be significant due to the highly peaked and localized nature of cortical sources; for electrodes located away from the source, the activity due to other cortical or even thalamic level sources might be present in sufficient amount to interfere with the recording of the desired information. It is for this reason that narrowly spaced electrodes located near the source should be used in recording cortical level sources while more widely spaced electrodes are desirable for deeper sources.

The Evoked Potential

The evoked potential is placed in the class of the 'event-related potentials' (ERP) that represents the whole group of recordable potentials in connection with a reference event determinable in time. The electrophysiological phenomena included in the previous definition can be divided into five classes: (1) sensorial evoked potentials, (a) acoustic, (b) somatic, (c) visual; (2) motor potentials, (3) long latency potentials relative to psycological complex variables; (4) slow potentials (CNV); (5) extracranial potentials.

With attention only to class 1a, in this paper we can affirm that an analysis made with the ERP aims at reaching three main goals: (1) to discern between the intracranial and the extracranial potentials; (2) to identify the anatomic locations of the biogenerators; (3) to determine the existing relationship between the ERP variations and the biogenerator activity.

The evoked potential aim, as stated above, is such that through it, theoretically, it is possible to receive information on the scalp coming from points of intracranial activity or lower, and to correlate those informations with behaviours and physio-pathological and psychological conditions of the subject. The location of these activating points is rather critical because of what we said previously about both the 'diffusion' due to the conductive volume and association zones to primary areas of generation.

The CNS elaborates manifold data coming from a large variety of receptors. It means that, as far the acoustic evoked responses are considered, figure 1 is extremely simple concerning block 3 and the links between this and block 2 particularly. From that we can deduce that the information given by the CNS is greatly modified from other blocks and also by the environment surrounding the subject. From this, as stated above, it follows that it is important to define and try to quantify, as much as possible, also the subject conditions and the environment during the evoked potential measurements.

Generally, the subject condition can be influenced by the following factors: environmental; physiological; specific; psychological. Among the psychological factors must be considered: attention; vigilance; assuefation; fatigue.

Conditions of Stimulation

Figure 5 shows an example of AEPs recorded by reference electrodes placed at the ear lobe and an exploring electrode at vertex ear distance [Bracale et al., 1971]. From a general point of view, in the AEPs it is possible to identify short latency (10–80 ms), medium latency (100–200 ms), and long latency (300–500 ms) responses. Generally the auditory stimulation is affected by modulating an acoustic carrier (of preselected tone) with a square wave length, t_0, and repetition, t, chosen by the operator.

Concerning the time, t, between one stimulus and the next one, we recall that from this depends the amplitude of the components N_1P_2 when the distance t between the next stimulus increases (fig. 5). Furthermore, it has been pointed out that utilizing a presentation of irregular, random or pseudo-random stimulation, we obtain evoked responses increasingly widen than those obtained with a regular presentation with the same frequency of the random condition (fig. 5) [Bracale et al., 1972].

Such a difference in the responses' amplitude lasts up to values of the interval between stimuli of 7–8 s. Beyond this interval, the responses from regular and irregular stimulation have the same amplitudes. The trend of experimental points suggested to try an interpolation by an exponential function is as follows:

$$A = B\,(1 - \exp\frac{t}{\tau}). \tag{4}$$

We considered the correctness of such an approximation from the standard deviation. In the interpolation we put at zero the value at the origin for the physiological consideration that a continuous tone (t = 0) does not produce evoked potentials. We have, also, to observe that the theoretical curve at the lower values of t loses importance from both physiological and mathematical points of view, because we cannot think that, as t decreases, the system under study could return to rest conditions after each stimulation.

At the computer, through the least square method, we looked for the B and t values minimizing the root-mean-square deviation and we found that such a curve really approaches in a satisfactory way the trend of experimental points. The curve obtained has been normalized to maximum value in order to make more comparable the tests made at a different time. In the following, we refer to some examples of such tests [Bracale et al., 1975].

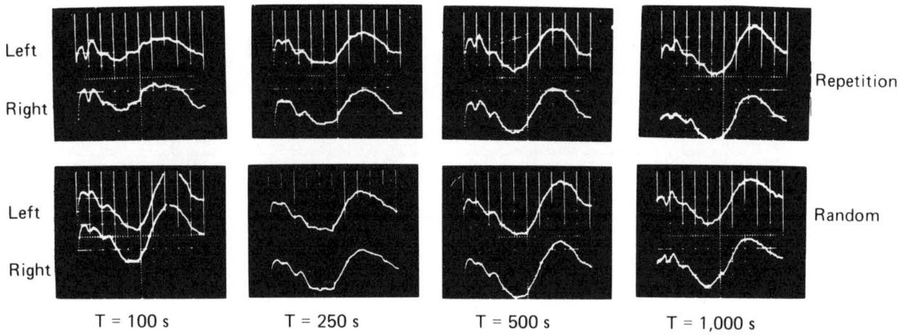

Fig. 5. Examples of AEP_S. Amplitude scale: points separated by 7 μV. Time scale: points separated by 20 ms. T = 100 t.

In figure 6 one can observe a remarkable coincidence between the obtained results from the right zone (curve a) and those from the left zone (curve b) of the subject M.B. The obtained values of the curve parameters are: (a) τ = 1.63 s ± SD 0.3; (b) τ = 1.82 ± SD 0.35.

Figure 7 shows the curve and the experimental values due to other tests made on the same subject but at a different time. The curve represents the average trend of all the tests, and from it one can find the uniformity on the value of the time constant τ.

The results of such research make some considerations possible: First of all the average time of presentation of 10 s between two successive stimuli assures the response's independency from the stimulation frequency. This time interval can be explained in metabolical terms as the time necessary to a complete return of excitability conditions of the various structures operating in the response-forming process. The attainment of this metabolical status of rest follows different temporal evolutions, also on affecting the equilibrium of the equation. Particularly, it could be interesting to investigate the causes of the time τ constant variability, for the purpose of a better definition of the patient 'status' (fig. 8).

The other variable from which the stimulation characteristics are depending is the duration t_0 of the signal impulse. This variable is directly connected to the stimulation signal spectrum.

As is known, the spectrum of the stimulation 'burst' is distributed around the sinusoidal carrier frequency with lobe lengths at $1/t_0$, except for the central one whose length is $2/t_0$. For example, with a tone at 1,000 Hz and a t_0 = 20 ms, a bandwidth of 100 Hz of the stimulating signal is rising at the central lobe. This means that in reality the subject is stimulated with a 'spurious' tone varying from 900 to 1,100 Hz. If the tone is at 125 Hz, with the same value of t_0, the subject will be stimulated with a sound presenting a spectrum from 75 to 200 Hz. Table I gives the bandwidth of the central lobe for values of t_0 varying from 10 to 80 ms.

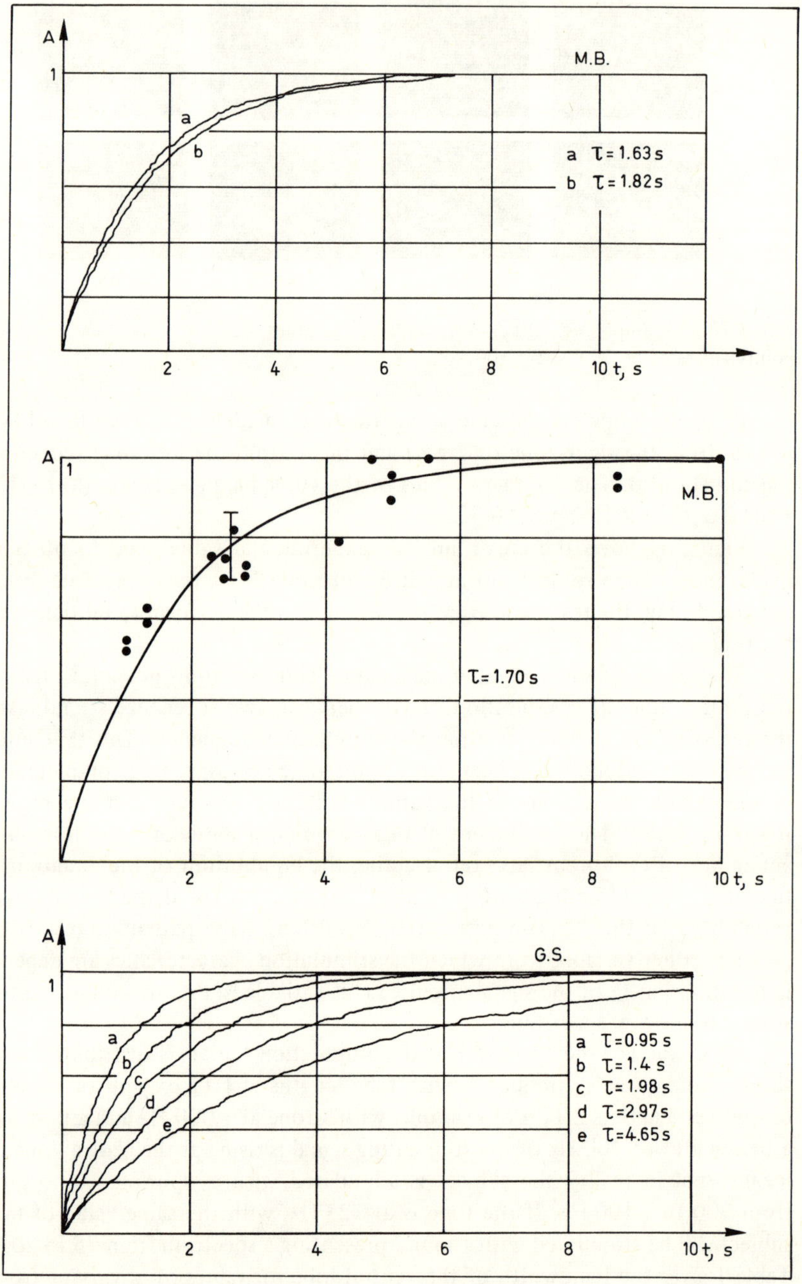
A
1
M.B.
a
b
a τ = 1.63 s
b τ = 1.82 s
2
4
6
8
10 t, s
A
1
M.B.
τ = 1.70 s
2
4
6
8
10 t, s
A
1
G.S.
a
b
c
d
e
a τ = 0.95 s
b τ = 1.4 s
c τ = 1.98 s
d τ = 2.97 s
e τ = 4.65 s
2
4
6
8
10 t, s

6

7

8

Fig. 6–8

Table I. Bandwidth of the central lobe for values of to varying from 10 to 80 msec. This lobe is the central one of the spectrum of the stimulation "burst" distributed around the sinusoidal carrier frequency.

t_0, ms	$2/t_0$, Hz
10	200
20	100
30	66
40	50
50	40
60	32
70	28
80	25

If we wish to keep constant the harmonic content, we should vary t_0 frequency by frequency and consequently, in order to stimulate always with the same energy, we should vary the bursts' amplitudes.

However, it is clear that such a condition is not convenient because the work would increase remarkably and the research would be more difficult. Then taking into account that generally we have to explore a frequency field from 250 to 6,000 Hz, it is possible to choose a constant value of t_0 for all tests, also for the lower frequency, in order to obtain a very small bandwidth percentage of the test.

A compromise value of t_0 is of 50 ms which, at 250 Hz, gives a bandwidth percentage of:

$$\frac{270-230}{250} \cdot 100 = 16\%. \tag{5}$$

The last equally important consideration to be taken into account is the number of successive stimulations. As is known, the evoked potential technique is based on the use of the mathematical technique of averaging. The use of information redundancy allows one to improve the signal/noise ratio according to:

$$S/N = \sqrt{n}, \tag{6}$$

Fig. 6. Example of interpolation by the exponential function (4) of the experimental point picked from the right zone (a) and those from the left zone (b) of the subject M.B.

Fig. 7. Experimental values fitted by (4), due to other tests made on the same subject M.B. but at a different time.

Fig. 8. Experimental values fitted by (4), due to tests made on a subject with different conditions of vigilance.

were n represents the number of stimuli and N represents noise; we compare every signal that is in a fixed phase with the stimulus itself. The spontaneous activity is also a part of this 'noise'. From the trend of the relationship we can deduce that we should use a great number of stimuli in order to improve remarkably the S/N ratio. This obviously is against pratical and physiological aspects. The latter particularly could cause a stress condition in the subject. This occurrence, at least, could affect the main hypothesis so that the evoked signal will stay steady enough during the whole period of analysis. In practice, the number of stimuli should not generally exceed 100. This, at worst, allows one to obtain an improvement of the S/N ratio of only 10 times. From that it follows, then, the necessity of preliminary technical improvements of the S/N ratio.

References

Bracale, M.; Scarpetta, G.; Serra, C.: Misura di potenziali evocati da stimolazione acustica; Rendiconti della LXXII Riunione. Annuale AEI, memoria 10.01, Venezia (1971).

Bracale, M.; Scarpetta, G.; Serra, C.: Problemi connessi al prelievo, all'elaborazione e all'interpretazione di potenziali evocati EEG; Annali Istituto Superiore di Sanità *8:* 714–718, Roma (1972).

Bracale, M.; Scarpetta, G.; Serra, C.: Parametri significativi dei potenziali EEG evocati da stimolazione acustica; Rivista di Neurologia, XLV *3:* 257–267 (1975).

Hoes, R.S.: An experimental and theoretical analysis of effects of volume conduction in a non-homogeneous medium on scalp and cortical potentials generated in the brain; PhD thesis, Milwaukee (1970).

M. Bracale, MD, Cattedra di Elettronica Biomedica, Instituto Elettrotecnico, Facoltà di Ingegneria, Via Claudio n. 21, I-80125 Napoli (Italy)

Adv. biol. Psychiat., vol. 6, pp. 165–172 (Karger, Basel 1981)

Toward a Neurochemical Interpretation of CNV in Psychiatry

Some Preliminary Results in Depressive Patients

M. Timsit-Berthier and M. Timsit

Laboratoire de Neurophysiologie clinique et de Psychopathologie, Liège, Belgique

Introduction

In earlier reports [*Timsit-Berthier* et al., 1969; *Timsit-Berthier,* 1976] about the use of contingent negative variation (CNV) in psychiatry, we pointed out a significantly more frequent occurrence of abnormal CNVs in both psychotic and neurotic populations, namely flat CNVs and long-lasting CNVs with post-imperative negative variation (PINV).

It was but an empirical assessment, based on electro-clinical correlations, and for which no explicate model was found. In the line of *Libet and Tosaka's* work [1970], *Marczynski* [1978] developed a neurochemical model of CVN based on data experimentally obtained in animals: he showed with this method that negative SPs and desynchronized EEG are mediated by a joined action of the cholinergic and catecholaminergic systems, while positive SPs and hypersynchronizing EEG result from a slackening in the tonus of catecholamines that allows the action of GABAergic hyperpolarizing circuits. This author found arguments favouring his model in the domain of psychopathology: schizophrenic patients, in whom a hyperactivity of the dopaminergic system would exist, display a pronolged CVN, whereas hyperactive children, who would suffer from a deficiency in the catecholaminergic system, display positive CVNs. *Marczynski's* [1978] model however does not refer to depressive patients, yet patients in whom modifications in the monoamines were described. On the one hand, there are abnormal features in the CVNs recorded in depressive patients [*Boltz* et al., 1979; *Timsit-Berthier,* 1976] and, on the other hand, CVN is modified in manic episodes in patients with bipolar depression [*Rizzo* et al., 1976]. These electro-clinical correlations have not been related yet with neurochemical data.

The present study precisely aims at assessing in depressive patients the validity of the neurochemical model of CNV proposed by *Marczynski* [1978], which achieves: (1) in establishing correlations between electrophysiological parameters (CNV, spectral analysis data) and diagnostic and syndromic categories, and (2) in studying the CNV changes induced by tricyclic antidepressive treatment (longitudinal study).

Methodology

1. Population

Among 54 depressive patients examined at our consultations since September 1978, 25 were selected on the following criteria: (a) presence of an ascertained depressive syndrome; (b) absence of any treatment at the time of consulting, (c) absence of manic episodes in the antecedents. 16 were consulting for the first time, 9 had been followed up for several years.

2. Electrophysiological Method

(a) Experimental Procedure. The patients received an uninterrupted block of about 100 stimuli pairs, in order to extract an artefact-free CNV, averaged over 48 trials. Each trial began with a warning 50-ms tone (S1), followed after 1 s by a series of flashes (S2), that the patient had to terminate by pushing a button with the right hand. The intertrial interval varied randomly between 10 and 30 s.

(b) Recording and Data Analysis. EEG (Cz, left ear lobe) and EOG (supra-infraorbital) were recorded with Ag/AgCl electrodes using amplifiers modified to yield a 5-s time constant. In addition, a bipolar recording (P3-P4) with TC = 0.3 s was preprocessed through a low-pass filter (33 Hz, 30 dB octave roll-off) and was analysed by the help of a fast Fourier transform (FFT) analysis. In order to quantify the level of arousal before S1 and the change of the EEG activity within the S1-S2 interval, the FFT analysis was performed twice: (a) during the second preceding S1 (spontaneous EEG without any stimulation); (b) during the second following S1 (S1-S2 interval of the CVN). Both analyses were then averaged on 48 trials.

(c) CNV and Spectral Power Measures. We measured: (a) CNV amplitude (voltage difference between 1-s pre-S1 baseline and 800–1000 ms post-S1 level); (b) P300 amplitude (voltage difference between 800 and 1000 ms post-S1 level, taken as baseline, and 300–500 ms post-S2 level), and (c) the reaction time. We also calculated the two following indexes of the power spectrum: the ratio percentage alpha/percentage theta + percentage delta for the spontaneous EEG (pre-S1 period), which is indicative of the general level of arousal, and the difference between alpha power before S1 and within the S1-S2 interval, which is indicative of the desynchronization versus hypersynchronization of the ongoing EEG during CNV (index % alpha 1–% alpha 2). This method has been described extensively [*Timsit-Berthier* et al., 1979].

3. Clinical Method

Initial clinical data were obtained through a psychiatric, non-directive interview and through a directive standardized interview [*Wing* et al., 1980] conducted by two different examiners. On the basis of these different data, the patients were classified in two groups, following *Winokur's* [1973] classification: primary unipolar depression (PD) and secondary depression (SD). It will be remembered that we eliminated subjects with a bipolar depression. In the patients given tricyclics, a retest, in the form of a second CNV and power spectrum recording, was performed 2–3 months after treatment onset. Quantitative data were submitted to one-way analysis of variance.

Table I. Characterization of the population under study according to the 3 types of CNV (normal, flat, prolonged)

CNV type	Subjects number	Age, years	Sex
Normal CNV	8	37.8 ± 12	7 F, 1 M
Flat CNV	9	37.5 ± 14	6 F, 3 M
Prolonged CNV	8	40.1 ± 11	7 F, 1 M

Table II. Electrophysiological parameters in the three groups of depressive patients. Patients of group II are characterized by a lower CVN amplitude, and diminished alpha reactivitiy. Patients of group III are characterized by a weak P 300 amplitude, corresponding to the prolongation of the CVN beyond 32

	CNV amplitude	P 300 amplitude	Reaction	$\frac{a}{\theta+\delta}$	a reactivity in S1–S2 interval
Normal CNV	22.2 ± 6.5	21.7 ± 5.9**	218.6 ± 46	1.36 ± 0.31	4.40 ± 2.44
Flat CNV	4.8 ± 4.48**	9.15 ± 5.42**	312 ± 168	1.07 ± 0.22	1.17 ± 1.65*
Prolonged CNV	16.56 ± 4.41	2.13 ± 4.50**	325 ± 106	1.23 ± 0.40	2.55 ± 2.46

** $p < 0.01$.

Table III. Clinical data related to the type of CNV. The central column gives the diagnosis (DG) following the psychiatric interview: PD stands for primary depression, SD for secondary depression. The last column presents mean total scores abtained at the present state examination (PSE): significantly lower scores are found in the group with normal CNVs

CNV type	DG	PSE total score
Normal CNV (8)	1 PD, 7 SD	21 ± 2.9**
Flat CNV (9)	8 PD, 1 SD	32 ± 9.8
Prolonged CNV (8)	4 PD, 4 SD	37 ± 8.9

** $p < 0.01$

Results

1. Electro-Clinical Correlations

Our subjects were divided into three groups according to the amplitude of their CNVs: we considered as 'normal' CNVs the curves for which the amplitude exceeded 10 μV, and the duration after S2 was inferior to 200 ms, as 'flat' CNVs, the curves with an amplitude inferior to 10 μV and a duration after S2 below 500 ms, and as 'prolonged' CNVs those with a duration superior to 500 ms [*Timsit-Berthier* et al., 1973]. The three groups so constituted comprised 8,9, and 8 subjects, respectively. Their characteristics are summarized in table I.

We felt the necessity to study, in a first approach, the distribution of reaction time and indexes derived from the spectral analysis among the three groups. The results obtained are illustrated by table II. It should be noticed that there is no correlation between the CNV parameters that we considered for classification of the subjects on the one hand, and the reaction time and the alpha/theta + delta index, on the other hand. There is however a significant ($p < 0.05$) correlation between a low CNV amplitude and a weak alpha reactivity during the interval between S1 and S2, as can be seen from the subjects in group II. Electro-clinical correlations are summarized in table III.

'Primary' depression characterizes the majority of subjects in group II, while 'secondary' depressions are mostly found in group I. Both types of depressions are equally represented in group III. The total score obtained at the PSE does not significantly differentiate between subjects of group II and III, those for whom, precisely, an 'abnormal' CNV is found. On the contrary, subjects of group I appear significantly different in this respect ($p < 0.01$). It should be noted that at a more elementary level PSE scores related to the following syndromes: 'slowness', 'general anxiety', 'situational anxiety', 'irritability', 'loss of interest and concentration' do not differentiate in a significant manner between subjects of groups II and III.

2. Longitudinal Study

We attempted to evaluate the changes that could be induced by a 2- to 3-month treatment with tricyclic antidepressive drugs at the level of two parameters of the CNV curves: the amplitude of the pre-imperative segment ('CNV'), and that of the post-imperative segment ('P300'). These measures were performed in only 13 of the patients, the others having either not received any antidepressive treatment (8 subjects) or been treated with benzamides (4 subjects).

The following results were obtained: In 11 patients out of 13, there is an increase of CNV amplitude following treatment with tricyclic antidepressants, and this whichever the group they belong to. What makes this phenomenon still more worth attention is the fact that, because of a process of habituation, CNV is known to decrease when recorded for the second time [*Timsit-Berthier* et al.,

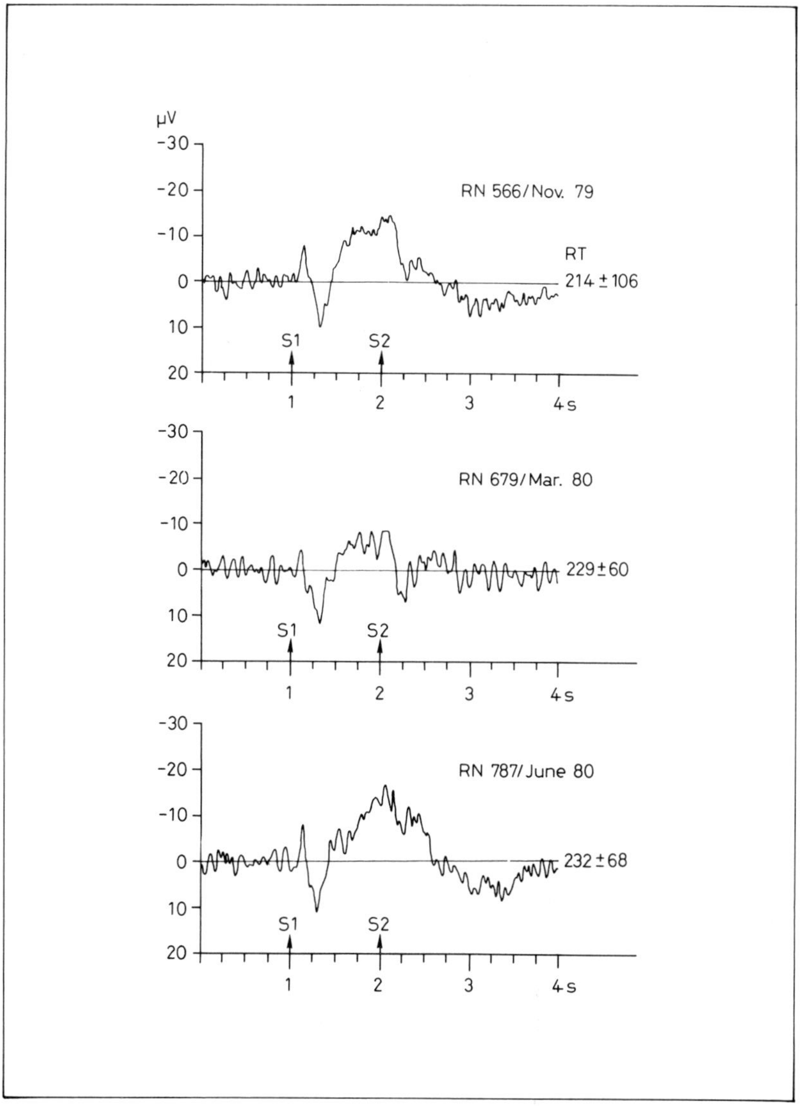

Fig. 1. Example of modifications in CNV amplitude under depressive condition. The patient is a woman aged 43. The top record was performed in the absence of any symptom and treatment of any kind. The middle record corresponds to a relapse and was done before onset of treatment. The bottom record follows a 3-month treatment with clomipramine (50 mg) and amitryptiline (50 mg).

1980]. P300 evolution is of a less unequivocal nature: while its amplitude decreases after treatment in the subjects with normal and flat CNVs (namely in 7 out of 9), it increases in a contrasting manner in 3 cases out of 5 in the subjects of the 'prolonged CNV' group. Figure 1 is representative of the drug effects observed on CNV and P300 amplitude. It shows a series of records in 1 patient of group II. The first one was performed when the patient was free of symptoms. The second one corresponds to a depressive relapse, and the third was realized after a 3-month treatment with tricyclic antidepressants.

To these electrophysiological data it is interesting to add some clinical considerations. The subjects with CNVs of normal amplitude rapidly showed a favourable evolution whatever treatment was given (psychopharmacology and/or psychotherapy). The subjects of group II proved particularly responsive to treatment with imipramine and nomifensine. The subjects of the third group proved extremely intolerant to tricyclic antidepressants like imipramine and nomifensine; it is also a highly interesting fact that the very same subjects remarkably responded to benzamides and/or amitryptiline treatment.

Discussion

Our starting project was to test *Marczynski's* [1978] hypothesis within the privileged framework of depression-suffering patients. Following this hypothesis, the patients with PD, who would present either a diminished metabolism of the catecholamines and/or 5-HT, or a diminished sensitivity of their receptors, would also have a low-amplitude CNV and a high-amplitude P300. On the other hand, the chronic treatment with tricyclics, which increases the metabolism of catecholamines and 5-HT, should also increase the amplitude of the CNV and decrease that of P300. The anticholinergic effects of such treatment were considered negligible as these tend to fade out after a few months.

Most of our results confirm these hypotheses: The patients suffering from PD electively display abnormal CNV with low amplitude, while the patients with SD exhibit a normal CNV. Under treatment with tricyclics, CNV increases in amplitude, and when the CNV is not prolonged, the P300 decreases. It is among the patients possessing a prolonged CNV that cases of intolerance to tricyclics are found. We can nevertheless indicate some elements that are contrary to those predicted by *Marczynski's* [1978] model: The presence of prolonged CNVs in patients with unipolar depression and showing no significantly more elevated anxiety scores when compared to the others. The reactivity of those prolonged CNVs display to tricyclic antidepressants, often resulting in an increase in the P300 amplitude.

To explain these phenomena, invoking the sole 'arousal level' notion [*Tecce* et al., 1978] seems to us difficult, as there is no correlation between the alpha/

theta + delta index and CNV amplitude [this was assessed on a sample of healthy volunteers; *Timsit-Berthier* et al., 1979]. It seems thus preferable to adopt a more dynamic model, such as the one proposed by *Howard* et al. [1980]. This model views the CNV as resulting from excitation and inhibition processes. It is at the level of inhibition phenomena that the serotoninergic system could be involved: on the one hand, it is implicated in depressive manifestations [*Van Praag*, 1980] and, on the other hand, it seems to play a role in habituation and drowsiness phenomena, which are known to provoke a polarity inversion of the CNV [*Timsit-Berthier* et al., 1980]. Under these conditions, prolonged CNVs in depressive patients would reflect a hypoactivity of the serotoninergic systems and/or receptors. As a concluding remark, we want to stress the interest such researches may bear for the physiologist, who focuses on the mechanismus underlying the CNV, and for the clinician, who has to make the best choice of an antidepressant.

Summary

The aim of this study is to test the neurochemical model of the contingent negative variation (CNV), developed by Marczynski and dealing with the role of cholinergic, catecholaminergic and GABAergic systems in the development of negative and positive shifts. We recorded, before treatment, the CNV of 25 depressive patients (13 primary and 12 secondary depressions). It appeared that CNVs with an amplitude superior to 10 μV and duration after S2 inferior to 200 ms characterized the majority of secondary depressions, while 'flat' CNVs, inferior to 10 μV and 'prolonged' CNVs with post-imperative negative variation (PINV) characterized the primary depressions. In the 13 subjects chronically treated with tricyclics, the amplitude of CNV increased and the amplitude of P300 tended to decrease. These data are discussed in relation to Marczynski's neurochemical model of the CNV.

Acknowledgments

We are indebted to Prof. *A. Dresse,* for welcoming us at the Pharmacology Department, and for the helpful advice that encouraged us to set up the present study. We also thank Mrs. *Scuvee-Moreau,* pharmacologist, who provided us with the necessary information to disentangle the complex neurochemical mechanism described in the model we used. We are grateful to Mrs. *Mantanus,* for statistical assistance, and to Mrs. *Magis* for gathering the documentation.

References

Bolz, J.; Giedke, H.; Heiman, H.: GSR, AEP and CNV in depressed patients and healthy controls; in Lehman, Callaway, Human evoked potentials applications and problems. Nato Conf. Series, Ser. III, p. 448 (1979).

Howard, R.; Fenton, G.W.; Fenwick, P.B.: Slow cerebral potentials in a 'go-no go' avoidance situation: a study on special hospital patients; in Barber, Evoked potentials, pp. 515–523 (University Park Press, Baltimore 1980).

Libet, B.; Tosaka, T.: Dopamine as a synaptic transmitter and modulator in sympathetic ganglia; A different mode of synaptic action. Proc. natn. Acad. Sci. USA *67:* 667–673 (1970).

Marczynski, T.J.: Neurochemical mechanisms in the genesis of slow potentials: a review and some clinical implications; in Otto, Multidisciplinary perspectives in event-related brain potential research, pp. 25–35. (US Government Printing Office, Washington 1978).

Rizzo, P.A.; Amabile, G.; Caporali, M.; Pierelli, F.; Spadaro, M.; Zanasi, M.; Moroccuti, C.: A longitudinal CNV study in a group of five bipolar cyclothymic patients. Biol. Psychiat. *4:* 581–586 (1976).

Tecce, J.J.; Savigno-Bowman, J.; Cole, S.O.: Drug effects on contingent negative variations and eyeblink: the distraction-arousal hypothesis; in Lipton, De Mascio, Killam, Psychopharmacology: a generation of progress, pp. 745–758 (Raven Press, New York 1978).

Timsit-Berthier, M.: La VCN et les maladies mentales. Acta psychiat. belg. *4:* 521–550 (1976).

Timsit-Berthier, M.; Delaung, J.; Konickx, N.; Rousseau, J.C.: Slow potential changes in psychiatry. 1. Contingent negative variation. Electroenceph. clin. Neurophysiol. *35:* 355–361 (1973).

Timsit-Berthier, M.; Gerono, A.; Rousseau, J.C.: CNV and functional state changes during long-lasting and repetitive recording sessions; in Kornhuber, Deecke, Motivation, motor and sensory processes of the brain: electrical potential behavior and clinical use. Prog. Brain Res. *54:* 673–681 (1980).

Timsit-Berthier, M.; Koninckx, N.; Dargent, J.; Fontaine, O.; Dongier, M.: Variations contingentes négatives en psychiatrie. Electroenceph. clin. Neurophysiol. *28:* 41–47 (1969).

Timsit-Berthier, M.; Rousseau, J.C.; Gerono, A.; Mantanus, H.: Etude comparée de la VCN et de l'EEG quantitatif au cours d'une tâche motrice simple. Rev. Electroencéphalogr. Neurophysiol. clin. *4:* 398–407 (1979).

Van Praag, H.M.: Central monoamine metabolism in depressions. I. Serotonin and related compounds. Compreh. Psychiat. *21:* 30–44 (1980).

Wing, J.K.; Cooper, J.E.; Sartorius, N.: Guide pour un examen psychiatrique. Traduit de l'anglais par Timsit-Berthier, Bragard-Ledent (Mardaga, Liège 1980).

Winokur, G.: The types of affective disorders. J. nerv. ment. Dis. *156:* 82–96 (1973).

M. Timsit-Berthier, Laboratoire de Neurophysiologie clinique et de Psychopathologie, 153, boulevard de la Constitution, B-4020 Liège (Belgium)

Adv. biol. Psychiat., vol. 6, pp. 173–179 (Karger, Basel 1981)

Differentiation of Depressive and Schizophrenic Psychoses by Evoked Potentials[1]

Charles Shagass, Richard A. Roemer, John J. Straumanis, Jr., Richard C. Josiassen[2]

Temple University Medical School and Eastern Pennsylvania Psychiatric Institute, Philadelphia, Pa., USA

Evoked potential (EP) studies of psychiatric populations have revealed many differences between patients and normal controls [*Shagass* et al., 1978a]. The largest and most consistent EP deviations from normal have been found in the major functional psychoses [*Shagass* et al., 1978b]. Although the fact that EPs of psychotics differ from those of normals and nonpsychotic patients is of great theoretical interest, EPs are more likely to find practical clinical application if they can help to discriminate between types of psychoses, such as schizophrenia and depression. Unfortunately, the EPs of patients with schizophrenic and affective psychoses have seldom been compared directly, because they differ in age and sex characteristics, for which they should be matched. Consequently, possible differences between the groups usually have been inferred from the ways in which each differed from matched normal controls; such inferential comparisons have generally suggested that their EPs are more alike than different [*Shagass* et al., 1978a]. Indeed, the similarities between the two groups led us to propose that the EP deviations reflect general functional alterations in psychosis that transcend nosology and are probably related to cognitive impairment [*Shagass* et al., 1978b].

The view that EPs of patients with schizophrenic and depressive psychoses do not differ requires modification in the light of results from a recent study, in which we were able to compare directly age- and sex-matched groups of psychotic depressives (mainly manic-depressive, depressed) and chronic schizophrenics [*Shagass* et al., 1980]. These patients were investigated with our comprehensive

[1] Research supported (in part) by USPHS Grant MH 12507.

[2] We thank the following for their assistance: *I.C. Hung, J. Kline, M. Kormanik, A. McGrath, W. Nixon, J. Pressman* and *S. Slepner*.

recording procedure, in which EPs evoked by four kinds of sensory stimuli are recorded from 15 locations [*Shagass* et al., 1977]. The direct comparisons revealed a large number of statistically significant differences between the EPs of the two psychotic groups. It then seemed appropriate to determine whether a relatively small number of EP measurements could be selected to provide effective discriminations between the schizophrenic and depressive psychoses. This paper reports our findings concerning such differential diagnostic indicators. It also presents a theoretical formulation, based on the EP findings, concerning the nature of information processing impairments in psychotic depression and chronic schizophrenia.

Methods

The basic recording procedures and the subject groups have been described in full elsewhere [*Shagass* et al., 1977, 1980]. The data come from comparisons between three groups of 16 subjects each, matched for age and sex: chronic schizophrenics, psychotic depressives, and nonpatient controls. A fourth group, nonpsychotic patients, was also studied, but their results are not shown. Ages ranged from 16 to 44 years (median, 30); there were 7 males and 9 females. The depressives were drawn from a larger group of 27 (fig. 1). Patients had been unmedicated for a median period of 10 days. Nearly all met the research diagnostic criteria of *Feighner* et al. [1972].

Electrode placements are shown in the head diagram of figure 1. Stimuli were: electrical pulses (0.1 ms duration, 10 mA above sensory threshold) over the left and right median nerves to elicit somatosensory EPs, designated as LSEP and RSEP, respectively; a checkerboard pattern flashed on a television screen for visual EPs (VEPs); binaural clicks for auditory EPs (AEPs).

EPs were compared in two ways: (a) by computing group mean EPs and performing t-tests between the consecutive corresponding data points, as in figure 1 [*Shagass* et al., 1977]; (b) by detecting consecutive peak amplitudes in key leads with a cursor program, and then using the latencies to compute amplitudes in the remaining leads [*Shagass* et al., 1980]; the amplitude values across leads were then subjected to multivariate profile analysis [*Morrison,* 1967] in order to detect group differences in amplitude and topography. EP peaks were designated by polarity (P, N) and usual latency (ms); thus, P30 denotes positivity 30 ms poststimulus. SEP peaks measured were: P15, N20, P30, P45, N60, P90, N130, P185, P290; VEP peaks were: N75, P90, N120, P200, P130, P300; AEP peaks were P30, P50, N75, P90, N110, P180, P360.

Results

Analyses were performed across all 14 EEG leads and, for SEP data, also for only the 5 leads (T3, T4 excluded) contralateral to the stimulated wrist. Schizophrenics had higher amplitudes than depressives for the following peaks: LSEP–N20, N60 (the more negative the higher the amplitude); RSEP–P15, P45; VEP–P200; AEP–P30. Depressives had higher amplitudes for: LSEP–P90 and N130;

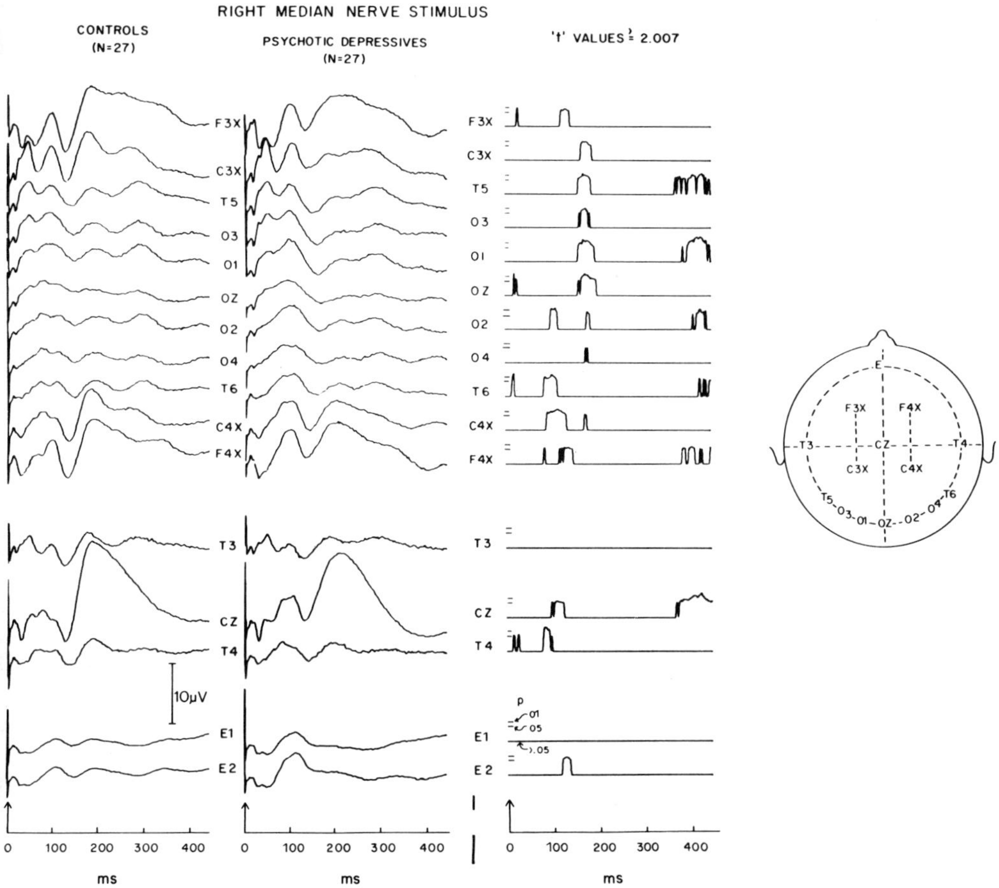

Fig. 1. Left and center columns: Mean SEPs to right median nerve stimuli of 27 controls and 27 psychotic depressive patients; 16 of each were matched for age and sex to schizophrenics. All leads referenced to linked ears; scalp positivity gives upward deflection. Right column gives results of two-tailed 't' tests performed on data points corresponding in time to those in EP tracings; 't' values under 2.007 were kept at baseline, while remainder were plotted according to magnitude, starting at an arbitrary level.

RSEP–P90, N130 and P185; VEP–P90. In addition, the topographies of LSEP N60, N130 and P185 and of RSEP N130 and P185 differed between the groups; N60 negativity extended more posteriorly in the schizophrenics, that of N130 extended more posteriorly in the depressives, and P185 positivity was maximal more anteriorly in the depressives.

Table I. Outline of SEP differences between psychotic depressives (PD), chronic schizophrenics (CS) and nonpatient controls (C) (n = 16 each Group)

	PD vs CS		PD vs C		CS vs C	
SEP Peak	PD	CS	PD	C	CS	C
P15		+		+		
N20		+				
P30						
P45		+			+	
N60		+			+	
P90	+		+			+
N130	+			+		+
P185	+			+		+
P290				+		+

Table II. Differentiation between 16 chronic schizophrenics (CS) and 16 psychotic depressives (PD) by selected measures

	Peak	Lead	Criterion	Number +/– PD	Number +/– CS	X^2	p
1 RSEP	P15	C3	> 0.90 μV	5/11	16/0	13.8	< 0.001
2	P45	01	> 3.25 μV	3/13	12/4	8.03	< 0.01
3	N130	03	< – 1.20 μV	6/10	13/3	4.66	< 0.05
4	P185	C4X, F4X	C4X > F4X	2/14	12/4	10.29	< 0.01
5 LSEP	N60	T6	negative	3/13	11/5	6.22	< 0.02
6	P90	CZ	< 4.61 μV	4/12	12/4	6.13	< 0.02
7	P185	C4X, F4X	C4X > F4X	3/13	10/6	4.66	< 0.05
				PD	CS		
		Sum of + (1–7)	0–3	16	1	24.60	< 0.001
			4–7	0	15		
		Sum of + (1–4)	0–2	15	1	21.13	< 0.001
			3–4	1	15		
		Sum of + (1–3)	0,1	14	0	21.46	< 0.001
			2,3	2	16		
		Sum of + (5, 6, 7)	0,1	13	3	10.13	< 0.01
			2,3	3	13		

Table I contrasts the depressives and schizophrenics with respect to SEP amplitude findings, a plus sign indicating higher amplitude. It will be seen that amplitudes of four early peaks, P15, N20, P45 and N60, were higher in the schizophrenics, while those of three later peaks, P90, N130 and P185, were greater in the depressives. Table I also outlines the results obtained by comparing each psychotic group with matched controls. Controls had higher amplitudes than depressives for all later peaks except P90, and also for P15; amplitudes of all later peaks were higher in controls than in schizophrenics, while the schizophrenics' P45 and N60 amplitudes were greater.

The results indicate that schizophrenics and depressives can be discriminated statistically be means of a large number of EP measurements. However, from a practical standpoint, the question is: How few measurements are needed to achieve a high level of differentiation? A retrospective analysis of the SEP data to answer this question yielded the results shown in table II. Seven SEP measures, each based on one or two leads, were selected; a criterion value, close to the median for the 32 patients, was determined and the values favoring the diagnosis of schizophrenia were designated as plus (+). The seven measures involved stimuli to both median nerves and recordings from 7 leads. While all individual measures discriminated ($p < 0.05$), a score (sum of plus values) based on all seven correctly classified 31 of the 32 patients. If only RSEP measures, derived from either 3 or 5 leads, were used, 30 of 32 patients would be classified correctly.

Discussion

Accurate differentiation between schizophrenic and depressive psychotics has assumed great importance as pharmacotherapies become more specific, and an objective aid to differential diagnosis would be clinically useful. Table II indicates that it may be possible to achieve a high level of discrimination between these psychotic groups by means of a relatively small number of SEP measures. Obviously, since the results are retrospective in nature, they require verification in a prospective study. The main point is that such differentiations are possible, and that they could be accomplished quite easily with a relatively simple procedure and equipment. The principal requirement now is an adequate body of data on well-diagnosed patients.

There are consistent findings indicating that early SEP components are of higher amplitude and less variable in chronic schizophrenics than in normals, while the reverse is true of later components; present SEP data are in agreement (table I). These findings formed the basis of a hypothesis that in chronic schizophrenia, there is impaired filtering of initial sensory inputs, reflected in higher amplitude and less variable early EPs, and that the impaired filtering alters later information processing, as indexed by lower amplitude, more variable later EPs [*Shagass,* 1976]. This hypothesis is, however, supported only by SEP and not by

VEP and AEP data [*Shagass* et al., 1979]. Present results indicate that, with respect to the contrast between early and late SEP components, psychotic depressives deviate from chronic schizophrenics in the same directions as do normals. This would suggest less impairment of the hypothesized filtering mechanism in depressives than in schizophrenics. On the other hand, the depressives did have lower than normal amplitude later EP components, except for P90; this reduction of later EP activity should index some impaired information processing. As will be seen, the temporal position of P90, at the center of the SEP peak sequence, may offer an explanatory clue about the nature of the impairment in depressives.

We have recently performed a study of selective attention in which SEPs were elicited by randomly stimulating the index and middle fingers of each hand; the subject was required to count one finger mentally. The counting condition produced not only the P400 wave [*Desmedt* et al., 1977] but also changes in all SEP components from P45 on. *Lavine* et al. [1980] have recently shown that even P30 is attention-sensitive. These findings suggest that SEP events can be modified by psychological factors at all levels of the sensory pathway; such effects would require the operation of filtering or modulating mechanisms at each level represented by the individual SEP components. Although our clinical SEP data were not obtained in a selective attention paradigm, the SEP characteristics can be taken to indicate the readiness of the underlying neural mechanisms to be engaged by a nonspecific probe stimulus. Our data suggest that filtering mechanisms are impaired at the earliest levels of the somatosensory pathway in chronic schizophrenics, and at a somewhat later level in psychotic depressives. Hence, SEP components prior to P90 are of higher amplitude in schizophrenics, and those from P90 on are diminished, while P90 is of higher than normal amplitude in psychotic depressives and later events are reduced.

Thus, we postulate that impaired filtering or modulation occurs in both major psychoses but at a later stage in psychotic depression than in chronic schizophrenia. Deficient information processing would result in both groups, but to a lesser extent in depression. This hypothesis should be more directly testable in studies comparing SEPs of patients with a selective attention paradigm like that of *Desmedt* et al. [1977].

Summary

To determine whether evoked potential (EP) indicators could differentiate between psychotic depressive and chronic schizophrenic patients, several kinds of EPs were compared in age- and sex-matched groups (N-16 each) of these patients and nonpatient controls. Retrospective analysis of the many EP differences between groups showed that seven somatosensory EP (SEP) measurements could classify correctly 31 of 32 schizophrenics and depressives; three SEP measures could detect 30 of 32. Possible clinical application of EPs in differential diagnosis of these psychoses is supported. A theoretical formulation is presented; it postulates that filtering mechanisms are impaired in both psychoses, but at different levels of the sensory pathway.

References

Desmedt, J.E.; Robertson, D.; Brunko, E.; Debecker, J.: Somatosensory decision tasks in man: early and late components of the cerebral potentials evoked by stimulation of different fingers in random sequences. Electroenceph. clin. Neurophysiol. *43:* 404–415 (1977).

Feighner, J.P.; Robins, E.; Guze, S.B.; Woodruff, R.A.; Winokur, G.; Munoz, R.: Diagnostic criteria for use in psychiatric research. Archs gen. Psychiat. *26:* 57–63 (1972).

Lavine, R.A.; Buchsbaum, M.S.; Schechter, G.: Human somatosensory evoked responses: effects of attention and distraction on early components. Physiol. Psychol. (in press, 1980).

Morrison, D.F.: Multivariate statistical methods (McGraw-Hill, New York 1967).

Shagass, C.: An electrophysiological view of schizophrenia. Biol. Psychiat. *11:* 3–30 (1976).

Shagass, C.; Ornitz, E.M.; Sutton, S.; Tueting, P.: Event related potentials and psychopathology; in Callaway, Tueting, Koslow, Event-related potentials in man, pp. 443–496 (Academic Press, New York 1978a).

Shagass, C.; Roemer, R.A.; Straumanis, J.J.; Amadeo, M.: Evoked potential correlates of psychosis. Biol. Psychiat. *13:* 163–184 (1978b).

Shagass, C.; Roemer, R.A.; Straumanis, J.J.; Amadeo, M.: Temporal variability of somatosensory, visual, and auditory evoked potentials in schizophrenia. Archs gen. Psychiat. *36:* 1341–1351 (1979).

Shagass, C.; Roemer, R.A.; Straumanis, J.J.; Amadeo, M.: Topography of sensory evoked potentials in depressive disorders. Biol. Psychiat. *15:* 183–207 (1980).

Shagass, C.; Straumanis, J.J.; Roemer, R.A.; Amadeo, M.: Evoked potentials of schizophrenics in several sensory modalities. Biol. Psychiat. *12:* 221–235 (1977).

Charles Shagass, MD, Eastern Pennsylvania Psychiatric Institute,
3300 Henry Avenue, Philadelphia, PA 19129 (USA)

Adv. biol. Psychiat., vol. 6, pp. 180–185 (Karger, Basel 1981)

Auditory Event-Related Potentials in Chronic Schizophrenics

Effects of Electrodermal Response Type and Demands on Selective Attention[1]

Rudolf Cohen, Werner Sommer, Max Hermanutz
University of Konstanz, Konstanz, FRG

It was not the aim of this study to identify certain components of event-related potentials (ERPs) that might allow a diagnostic discrimination of psychiatric patients superior to clinical interviews, nor was it our intent to elucidate neurophysiological abnormalities pathognomonic of schizophrenia [*Shagass* et al., 1978]. Our primary interest was rather to explore whether available knowledge about the psychological processes intimately related to late components of the ERP [*Donchin* et al., 1978] might provide some insight into pecularities of information processing prevalent among chronic schizophrenics and especially among those 40–50%, who – according to an impressive series of studies [*Venables*, 1977] – do not show any changes in electrodermal activity to stimuli that normally elicit an orienting response. Do these patients also differ from others in their auditory ERPs, and do such differences depend on the task-relevance of the stimuli? Since several studies have also reported deficiencies in the habituation of those schizophrenics who exhibit electrodermal responses and in view of the challenging studies of *Steffy and Galbraith* [1980] on 'redundancy-associated deficits' in the reaction times of chronic schizophrenics, we systematically varied the number of non-signal stimuli preceding the ERP-eliciting events. All 'significant' results reported here have to be considered preliminary in nature, because the number of possible comparisons is rather high.

[1] We wish to express our deep appreciation to the staff and the patients of the Psychiatrisches Landeskrankenhaus Reichenau.

Method

Subjects were 22 healthy employees, 22 chronic alcoholics and 25 chronic non-paranoid schizophrenics from a German psychiatric state hospital. Alcoholics had been abstinent for at least 3 weeks and were off tranquilizers; 22 of the schizophrenics were receiving maintenance dosages of neuroleptics. Psychiatric classification was based on the consensus of two experienced psychiatrists in line with DSM III [1980] criteria, who also assessed the patients on the brief psychiatric rating scale (BPRS) [*Overall and Gorham,* 1976]. Median duration of hospitalization was 8 months for alcoholics and 4.4 years for schizophrenics. All subjects were male; groups were matched for age (median = 41 years) and educational status.

To determine the electrodermal response type, 15 tones (75 dB, 1,000 Hz, 1 s, 25 ms rise time) were presented at intervals varying from 25 to 40 s. Skin conductance was recorded with a Beckman constant voltage system (Ag/AgCl electrodes, 0.5% Hellige isotonic jelly). Subjects were defined as non-responders (NR), habituators (H) or non-habituators (NH), depending on whether they showed no responses greater than 0.05 μmho to three consecutive stimuli at the very beginning, later in the series, or whether this criterion was not reached across the 15 stimuli. All subjects showed shifts of skin conductance in the social exchange before and after the experiment proper.

For the ERPs, rare (70 dB SL) and frequent (50 dB SL) clicks of 0.1 ms (ISI = 1.65 s) were presented in a ratio of 10:90. Rare clicks were separated by 4–12 frequent clicks. A set of light bars was presented with the same temporal distribution as the rare clicks on a screen concomitantly with some of the frequent clicks. In counterbalanced order subjects had to count either the rare clicks or the visual stimuli until 61 artefact-free ERPs to rare clicks could be averaged on-line or until 75 rare clicks had been presented. The EEG was recorded with Ag/AgCl electrodes at Fz, Cz, Pz and from above the left eye referred to linked mastoids (bandpass: 0.05–70 Hz; roll-off: 6 dB/octave). Sampling at 200/s was done for 800 ms starting 50 ms before stimulus onset. Trials with EOG excursions greater than 60 μV were discarded. The covariance matrices of the ERPs to rare and frequent clicks were submitted to separate PCAs, the resulting factor scores to separate Anovas with degrees of freedom corrected according to *Greenhouse and Geisser* [1959]. Three components were analysed for ERPs to rare clicks (80.7% total variance), four components for ERPs to frequent clicks (71.4% total variance). The Newman-Keuls procedure was used for a posteriori tests ($p < 0.05$), the Mann-Whitney test for non-parametric comparisons.

Results and Discussion

ERP factor scores from rare clicks (fig. 1b) are smaller in schizophrenics than in alcoholics or normals, both for a slow negative shift (N220) with peak amplitude at 220 ms ($F[2.66] = 4.04$; $p < 0.05$) and for the P340 component ($F[2.66] = 6.55$; $p < 0.01$). This reduction in amplitudes of late components is in line with many earlier findings [*Roth* et al., 1979; *Shagass* et al., 1978]. Differences between groups in P340 amplitudes (fig. 1d) are more pronounced when the ERP-eliciting clicks had to be counted than when they were irrelevant for the task ($F[2.66] = 8.30$; $p < 0.01$). Counting clicks also increases N90 amplitudes of non-target clicks in normals and alcoholics but leads to a paradoxical decrease in schizophrenics at Cz and Pz ($F[2.66] = 3.87$; $p < 0.05$). Apparently,

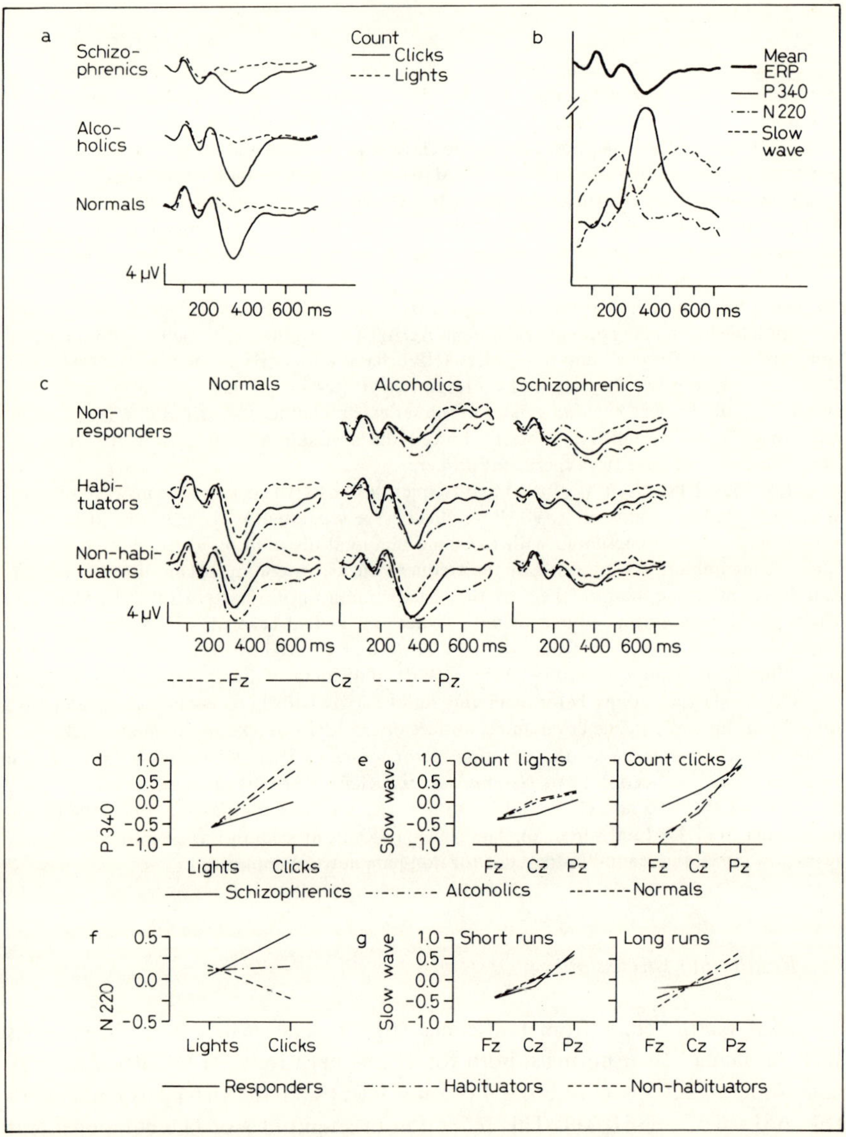

Fig. 1. ERPs to rare clicks from schizophrenics (S), alcoholics (A) and normals (N). *a* Across-subject vertex ERPs for Ss, As and Ns when rare clicks or lights were counted. *b* Super-average ERP (across all subjects, leads and experimental conditions) and loading for the varimax-rotated factors extracted by principal components analysis. *c* Across-subjects ERPs to target clicks from Fz, Cz and Pz for Ss, As and Ns, separated according to electrodermal response type. *d* Mean P340 score for Ss, As and Ns when rare clicks of lights were

the instruction to focus attention was more likely to produce interferences on the part of the schizophrenics rather than to activate selective filter mechanisms. Whether or not the smaller amplitudes of the later components are a result of increased latency jitter [*Roth* et al., 1979], they most likely reflect an increased variability in attention and compliance with the task [*Callaway,* 1975]: the deviation from the correct count of target clicks is greater ($z \geqslant 4.34$, $p < 0.01$) for schizophrenics (median = 20.0%) than for alcoholics (median = 3.5%) and normals (median = 3.0%). Their counting performance is correlated ($rho \leqslant 0.59$, $p < 0.01$) both with the P340 score for target clicks and with its difference between the two tasks ($rho \leqslant 0.58$, $p < 0.01$). Neither the N220 nor the P340 component correlates with medication dose [*Haase,* 1977] or BPRS scales ($-0.19 \leqslant rho \leqslant -0.04$). Only the difference between the tasks in N90 amplitude correlates ($rho \leqslant 0.37$, $p < 0.05$), with the BPRS activation scale.

The slow wave (SW) for rare clicks shows differences between groups in interaction with task ($F[2.66] = 4.12$; $p < 0.05$), and lead ($F[2.66] = 3.82$; $p < 0.05$): Counting the ERP-eliciting clicks increases the parietal positivity for all groups (fig. 1e), but the concomitant increase of the frontal negativity found in normals and alcoholics is virtually absent in schizophrenics. This finding might be seen as related to the low cerebral blood flow in frontal regions of chronic schizophrenics reported by *Franzén and Ingvar* [1975]. The smaller the frontal SW to target clicks, the higher the total BPRS score ($rho \leqslant 0.43$, $p < 0.05$) and the subscales anxiety/depression ($rho = 0.41$), anergia ($rho = 0.42$) and though disturbance ($rho = 0.37$). The corresponding correlations for the parietal SW are negligible ($-0.09 \leqslant rho \leqslant 0.08$). However, the positivity of the SW at vertex is correlated with counting performance ($rho = 0.38$, $p < 0.05$), possibly reflecting prolonged stimulus processing in some of the schizophrenic subjects. None of the SW scores are correlated with level of medication ($rho \leqslant 0.21$).

Well in line with the literature [*Venables,* 1977], 10 of the 25 schizophrenics were classified as electrodermal NRs, 6 as Hs and 9 as NHs. Among the 22 alcoholics there were 4 NRs, 8 Hs and 10 NHs. Because there were no NRs among the 22 normals (14 appeared as NHs), comparisons between electrodermal response types (EDT) were confined to the two groups of patients. The three types did not differ with respect to age, education, length of hospitalization,

---

counted. *e* Mean slow wave scores from Fz, Cz and Pz for Ss, As and Ns when rare clicks or lights were counted. *f* Mean N220 scores for electrodermal non-responders, habituators and non-habituators (normals excluded) when rare clicks or lights were counted. *g* Mean slow wave scores from Fz, Cz and Pz for electrodermal non-responders, habituators and non-habituators (normals excluded) when rare clicks followed short (4–8) or long (9–12) runs of frequent clicks.

medication or any of the BPRS scales ($0.12 \leq F[2.41] \leq 2.24$). As usual skin conductance level ($F[2.41] = 6.47$; $p < 0.01$) and number of spontaneous fluctuations ($F[2.41] = 16.54$; $p < 0.01$) were lower in NRs than in Hs and NHs. Counting performance was slightly but insignificantly worse in Hs (median = $14.0\%_{dev}$) than in NHs (median = $8.0\%_{dev}$) and NRs (median = $5.5\%_{dev}$).

There were no differences between the EDTs as main effects or in interaction with diagnostic group for the $\overline{P300}$ components for either the rare or the frequent clicks. Differences were only found for the slow negative shift (N220) and the SW from the rare clicks. Figure 1f depicts the interaction task × EDT ($F[2.41] = 4.12$; $p < 0.05$) for the N220 component. While the factor scores appear unaffected by task demands for the Hs and show an increase in negativity for NHs when clicks were to be counted, this task leads to a significant decrease for the NRs. This paradoxical diminution of a component closely related to processes of target detection [*Näätänen and Michie,* 1979] in the NRs might be seen as functionally corresponding to the lack of electrodermal responses and interpreted as manifestation of inhibitory processes produced by the instruction to attend. Since N220 scores and their differences between tasks do not correlate with counting performance ($rho \leq -0.12$), one might conclude that the elicitation of these inhibitory processes can be as effective for target apperception as those processes which in normals and NHs produce an enhancement of the N220 component.

An interaction between EDT and group ($F[2.41] = 3.73$; $p < 0.05$) shows the SW to rare clicks to be more negative for alcoholic than for schizophrenic NRs ($p < 0.01$). This interaction is embedded in a fourfold interaction with task and lead ($F[2.41] = 4.44$; $p < 0.05$), which could not be decomposed into more simple effects. The frontally rather unresponsive SW of schizophrenics is most reduced in that electrodermal response type which is found mainly in schizophrenics, the NRs. As depicted in figure 1g, the length of the preceding run of frequent clicks affects the SW differently depending on EDT ($F[2.41] = 5.31$; $p < 0.01$): Following short runs of 4–8 frequent clicks, NHs show a smaller parietal positivity to rare clicks than both Hs and NRs. This might reflect some advantage of the NHs in handling rare events following up to 8 frequent clicks. After longer series with 9–12 frequent clicks the NRs show a reduction both in the frontal (significant only in the comparison with the NHs) and the parietal part of the SW. Apparently, NRs not only give evidence of paradoxical inhibition in processes related to target apperception but also an attenuation of brain activities related to later stages of information processing when the stimuli occur against a highly monotonous background; this accords well with the notion of a 'redundancy-associated deficit' in chronic schizophrenics [*Steffy and Galbraith,* 1980]. Except for these interactions, neither diagnostic group nor electrodermal type modified the effects of serial order on the ERPs to frequent and rare clicks [*Hermanutz* et al., 1980].

Summary

Chronic schizophrenics, alcoholics and normals were compared in their ERPs to rare and frequent clicks, when either the rare clicks or interspersed light stimuli had to be counted. Schizophrenics but not alcoholics have reduced amplitudes both of the N90 component for frequent clicks and of an early negative shift (N220), the P340 component, and the frontal negativity of the slow wave for rare clicks. In schizophrenics P340 amplitude is correlated with counting performance, the frontal negativity of the slow wave inversely related to ratings of psychopathology. Electrodermal nonresponders among patients show a paradoxical decrease in N220 amplitude when the ERP-eliciting clicks were to be counted and an attenuation of the slow wave if the rare clicks followed long series of frequent clicks.

References

Callaway, E.: Brain electrical potentials and individual psychological differences (Grune & Stratton, New York 1975).

Donchin, E.; Ritter, W.; McCallum, W.C.: Cognitive psychophysiology: the endogenous components of the ERP; in Callaway, Tueting, Koslow, Event-related brain potentials in man, pp. 349–441 (Academic Press, New York 1978).

Diagnostic and statistical manual of mental disorders (DSM III) (Am. Psychiatric Association, Washington 1980).

Franzén, G.; Ingvar, D.H.: Absence of activation in frontal structures during psychological testing of chronic schizophrenics. J. Neurol. Neurosurg. Psychiat. *38:* 1027–1032 (1975).

Greenhouse, S.W.; Geisser, S.: On methods in the analysis of profile data. Psychometrika *24:* 95–112 (1959).

Haase, H.J.: Therapie mit Psychopharmaka und anderen seelisches Befinden beeinflussenden Medikamenten (Schattauer, Stuttgart 1977).

Hermanutz, M.; Cohen, R.; Sommer, W.: The effects of serial order in long sequences of auditory stimuli on event related potentials. Psychophysiology (in press).

Näätänen, R.; Michie, P.T.: Different variants of endogenous negative brain potentials in performance situations: a review and classification; in Lehmann, Callaway, Human evoked potentials: applications and problems, pp. 251–267 (Plenum Press, New York 1978).

Overall, J.E.; Gorham, D.R.: 047 BPRS. Brief psychiatric rating scale; in Guy, ECDEU assessment manual for psychopharmacology, pp. 157–169 (Rev. Ed., Rockville 1976).

Roth, W.T.; Horvath, T.B.; Pfefferbaum, A.; Tinklenberg, J.R.; Mezzich, J.; Kopell, B.S.: Late event-related potentials and schizophrenia; in Begleiter, Evoked brain potentials and behavior, pp. 499–516 (Plenum Press, New York 1979).

Shagass, C.; Ornitz, E.M.; Sutton, S.; Tueting, P.: Event-related potentials and psychopathology; in Callaway, Tueting, Koslow, Event-related brain potentials in man, pp. 443–509 (Academic Press, New York 1978).

Steffy, R.A.; Galbraith, K.: Relation between latency and redundancy-associated deficit in schizophrenic reaction time performance. J. abnorm. Psychol. *89:* 419–427 (1980).

Venables, P.H.: The electrodermal psychophysiology of schizophrenics and children at risk for schizophrenia: controversies and developments. Schiz. Bull. *3:* 28–48 (1977).

Prof. Dr. R. Cohen, Sozialwissenschaftliche Fakultät, Fachgruppe Psychologie der Universität Konstanz, Postfach 5560, D-7750 Konstanz 1 (FRG)

Adv. biol. Psychiat., vol. 6, pp. 186–194 (Karger, Basel 1981)

Evoked Potential Measures of Attention and Psychopathology

M.S. Buchsbaum, R. Coppola, E.S. Gershon, D.P. Van Kammen, J.I. Nurnberger
Biological Psychiatry Branch, NIMH, Bethesda, Md., USA

Introduction

Deficits in attention have been widely reported in both schizophrenia [*Garmezy,* 1978] and childhood hyperactivity [*Douglas,* 1972]. These results, more consistent than many neurochemical findings, have led many theorists to view attention disorders as fundamental and to suggest that the neurochemical and electrophysiological mechanisms of attention may provide a key for understanding these illnesses [*Matthyssee,* 1978].

In psychiatric patients, many different features of the attentional processes have been reported to be deficient, including selective attention, vigilance and switching attentional sets. Abnormalities of the motor system itself, including elevations in creatinine phosphokinease and pathological muscle fibers have been reported [*Meltzer,* 1979], and EMG studies of schizophrenics' reaction time [*Schneider and Grossi,* 1979] suggest that peripheral factors may be important in differences previously held to be due solely to central dysfunction.

The evoked potential technique seems particularly appropriate for separating differing central and peripheral attentional factors and for localizing attentional deficits in particular cortical areas. Of all of the EP components, the N120 appears most closely linked to selective attention. The amplitude of N120 appears to index the process by which 'stimuli are selected or rejected on the basis of their simple physical attributes' [*Schwent* et al., 1976, p. 313]. The relationship between the N120 and attention is reviewed elsewhere [*Hillyard* et al., 1978].

The literature on N120 in schizophrenia has tended to reveal smaller N120 than normal controls even when an attentional task was uncontrolled [see reviews by *Shagass* et al., 1978; *Buchsbaum,* 1979]. But studies have differed in EEG lead derivation, patient medication status, and whether N120 was measured relative to a baseline or confounded with P100 or P200 variation. In this review of a series of NIMH studies, we have focused on the N120 component, comparing differences observed between off medication schizophrenics and normal controls with the effects of an attention-enhancing drug, amphetamine. Further results applying topographic techniques to the N120 component will illustrate the problems inherent in interpreting EP data from only 1 or 2 EEG leads.

Methods

Evoked Potential Stimuli and Recording

The stimuli were four intensities of light flashes, and four intensities of tones each presented 64 times in a randomized sequence. Each stimulus was 500 ms long followed by a 500-ms interstimulus interval. The light flashes were viewed on a transluscent screen, rear illuminated by flourescent tubes under computer control [*Coppola*, 1977]. Auditory stimuli were four intensities of 1,000 Hz tones similarly presented using a computer-controlled oscillator at 50, 60, 70 and 80 dB through two loudspeakers in an acoustically attenuated room (background less than 20 dB at 1,000 Hz; less than 2 dB variation in the cubic foot surrounding the subject's head.) The stimuli were presented in a pseudorandom sequence so that each intensity of light and tone was preceded by every other tone or light an equal number of times.

For the assessment of attentional enhancement, all subjects first received training in the correct identification of the intensity of the visual and auditory stimuli [*Schechter and Buchsbaum*, 1973]. Subjects were then given three different tasks in random order: (1) light attention (LA), counting the number of visual stimuli which were of the same intensity in a row, ignoring intervening tones; (2) tone attention (TA), counting the number of tones similarly ignoring lights, and (3) mental arithmetic (MA), subtracting seven serially from 2,000. For each condition, the same EP sequence of lights and tones was presented. The schizophrenic patients received only the LA and TA tasks.

EEG was recorded from left and right temporoparietal leads [the center of a triangle P_3-T_3-T_5, termed W_3; *Matsumiya* et al., 1972] amplified (3 dB points 0.3 and 110 Hz) analogue-filtered and digitized at 250 samples/s in the first series of experiments.

Statistical analysis included two-way and three-way Anova with repeated measures and trend effects for intensity and t-tests on the mean of the lowest two intensities [to match data in *Buchsbaum* et al., 1978]. To assess attentional differences, the EP amplitude during condition TA was subtracted from LA; positive numbers for the difference score thus give the increase in amplitude with selective attention. For the cortical mapping experiments, Grass P511 amplifers were used. EPs were first detrended using linear regression and then digitally filtered to remove frequencies below 4 Hz and above 30 Hz as described (with a different bandpass) elsewhere [*Lavine* et al., in press]. Eye movements and artifacts were monitored using lead Fp_1; trials exceeding a threshold were automatically excluded from the average for all leads. Individuals exceeding a 50% trial loss on any condition were excluded (one individual). For the cortical maps, in addition to the 12 electrodes normally on the left side (10–20 system) or midline (F_Z-C_Z-P_Z-O_Z), four additional electrode locations were added to provide greater resolution of the posterior cortex. These are placed at the centers of squares formed by connecting P_3-P_2-O_Z-O_1 (PO), C_3-C_Z-P_Z-P_3 (CP) T_3-C_3-P_3-T_5 (TCP) and F_7-F_3-C_3-T_3 (FTC). The 16 values were then used to interpolate values over the entire scalp area as described elsewhere. EPs were measured as described elsewhere [*Buchsbaum* et al., 1977]; only the N120 area integration results are presented here (116–152 ms).

Patients and Normal Controls

A sample of 26 patients who met research diagnostic criteria [*Spitzer* et al., 1975] for schizophrenia or schizoaffective illness (17 males and 9 females, mean age 26) and who were hospitalized on an inpatient research unit served as subjects. 26 normal nonpatient volunteers, age- and sex-matched, served as controls. For studies with amphetamine, 17 pairs of monozygotic and dizygotic twins (mean age 25) were studied [*Nurnberger* et al., 1980]. Placebo or 0.3 mg/kg dextroamphetamine was administered intravenously in random order on separate days.

Results

Effects of Amphetamine in Normal Volunteer Twins

Amphetamine enhanced mean visual N120 amplitude (across the four intensities) for the left temporoparietal lead most (0.99 μV) when subjects attended to the lights (fig. 1), two-way drug by intensity Anova, drug effect ($F = 17.05$, d.f. = 1.33, $p < 0.001$), moderately (0.80 μV) when they attended to tones ($F = 4.94$, $p < 0.05$) and slightly (0.62 μV) when they did mental arithmetic ($F = 2.96$, n.s.). These effects, while greater at low than high intensity stimulation, did not interact significantly with intensity (treatment $\times$ intensity interaction).

Amphetamine enhanced the attentional increase in N120 amplitude, but this effect was restricted to the low intensities, where the only significant attentional effects were seen. The overall drug by intensity by task Anova did not reach significant levels for the left temporoparietal lead, but individual t-tests for the mean of the lowest two intensitites did ($t = 2.24$, $p < 0.05$, light attention – tone attention, fig. 2). It should be noted that a significant attention effect itself was only confirmed for the low-intensity stimulus, amphetamine condition in this sample (+0.43 μV, $t = 2.15$).

Test-retest reliability was available for 15 subjects, one member of each pair, who received amphetamine twice, 1 or more weeks apart. For the mean of the two lowest intensities, the test-retest correlation was light attention 0.74, tone attention 0.62, and mental arithmetic 0.34.

Schizophrenics versus Normals (fig. 3)

When all 26 schizophrenics' EPs were compared to all normals, no significant group by task or group $\times$ task $\times$ intensity interaction emerged for visual EP N120. However, on examination of the EPs recorded during light attention, the lowest two intensities revealed a significantly smaller amplitude, consistent with previous findings (2.07 vs 2.68 μV, $t = 1.80$, $p < 0.05$, 1-tailed). Male nonschizoaffective patients ($n = 11$) were the only group in which the hypothesized attentional deficit was clearly confirmed for light-attention-tone attention differences (normals, +0.58 μV increase with attention, schizophrenics, –0.18 μV; $t = 1.85$, $p < 0.05$, 1-tailed).

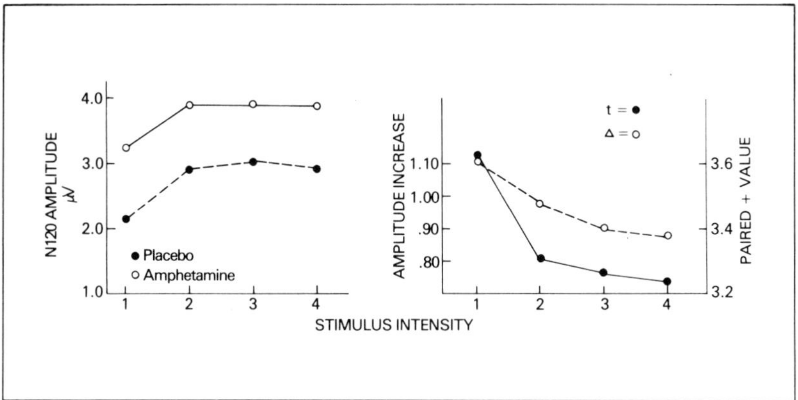

1

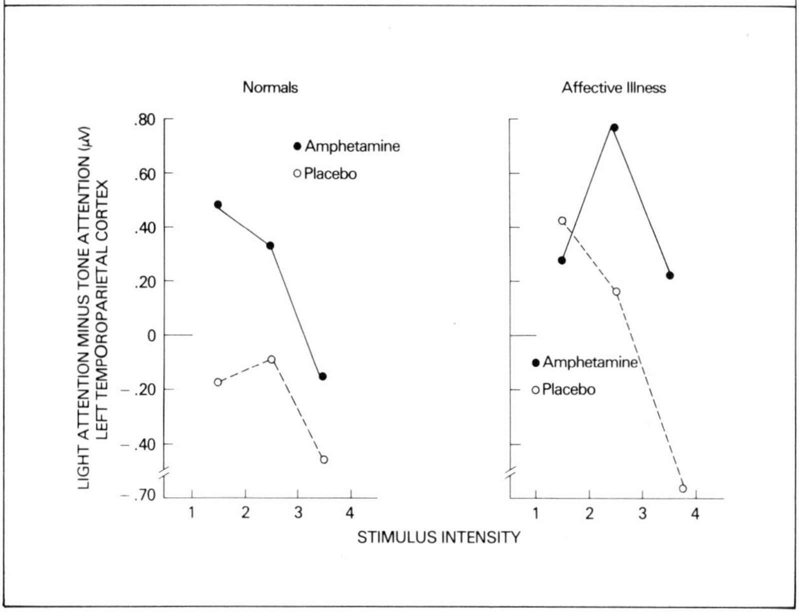

2

Fig. 1. Effect of amphetamine (0.3 mg/kg, i.v.) on visual EPs, N120 component, left temporoparietal cortex, in 34 adult twins doing a visual cognitive task. *a* EP amplitude after placebo and amphetamine administration. *b* t-values for amphetamine effect and amphetamine-induced amplitude increase. Note trend for greater effect at low intensity, which becomes more dramatic when attentional enhancement is calculated (fig. 2).

Fig. 2. a Comparison with similarly collected data on 9 patients with affective disorder [*Reuss* et al., 1979]. *b* Visual EP attention enhancement by amphetamine in 34 normal adult twins for N120. The ordinate shows the difference in microvolts between the visual EP amplitude while subjects attended to light stimuli, and while they attended to tone stimuli. Consistant with other reports, attention effects were greater for low intensity stimuli.

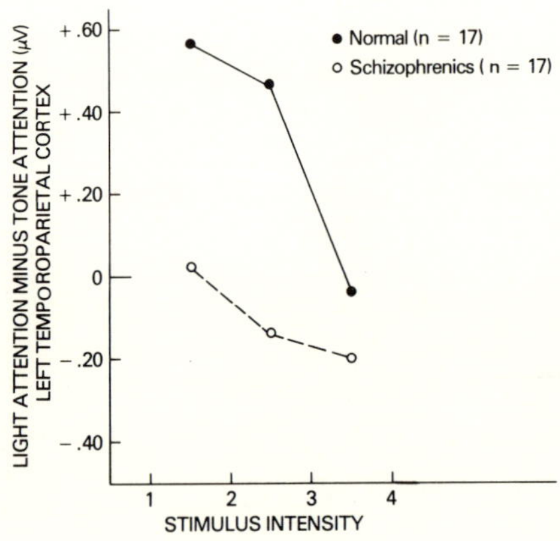

Fig. 3. Visual EP amplitude enhancement (N120, left temporoparietal cortex) in 17 normal adults and 17 male schizophrenics. Again, as for the drug effect (fig. 2), the greatest difference is seen for the lowest intensity. The normals, but not the schizophrenics, showed significant attention effects. The group differences in attentional effects were confirmed by two-way Anova on attentional differences (group by intensity interaction, $F = 4.93$, linear trend effect, 1, 32 d.f., $p < 0.05$).

Topographic Maps of Visual EPs and Attention

7 subjects received the attentional paradigm with the 16-lead recording technique. Figure 4 shows the comparison of topographic patterns derived from EPs recorded in resting non-attending subjects with the EP attentional enhancement effect. The N120 mean amplitude has both a frontal and occipital component with relatively low levels in the temporal and parietal areas. The attention effect (light attention minus tone attention) shows a frontal and posterior parietal distribution. T values for t-tests done between N120 amplitude at low intensity for the light attention and tone attention conditions at each of the 16 leads are mapped using the same procedure (fig. 5).

1 schizophrenic patient had the topographic mapping applied to data collected during the attention paradigm. His posterior parietal areas show no attentional increases in N120, quite distinct from the group of 7 normal subjects.

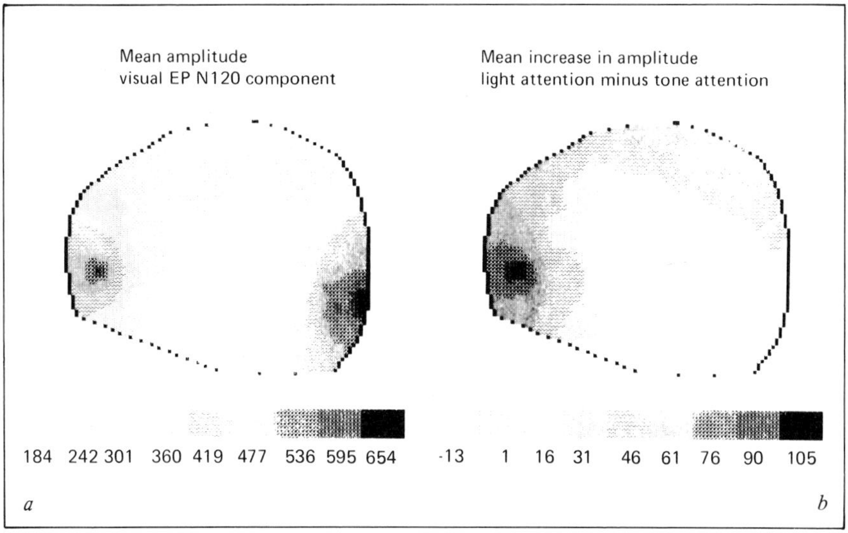

Fig. 4. Topographic maps of scalp distribution of N120 component, showing left hemisphere frontal cortex on the left. Scale in microvolts × 100. ***a*** Mean amplitude of N120 across four intensities shows frontal and occipital pole maximum, resembling 126 msec map of ***Ragot and Remond*** [1978] and ***Lehmann and Skrandies*** [1980]. ***b*** Mean difference between visual N120 amplitude recorded while subjects do a visual cognitive task and while subjects do a auditory task. Most areas of the scalp distribution are positive, indicating EP amplitude is larger during selective attention to the visual stimulus. Frontal and posterior parietal cortex show the greatest attentional enhancement; temporal cortex is the lowest.

Discussion

The test-retest reliability, sensitivity to drugs known to enhance attentional performance, and specific cortical distribution support the use of the N120 component in clinical studies of attention dysfunction. The finding of diminished EP attentional enhancement with task is certainly consistant with a wide body of cognitive studies of schizophrenia. The opposite directions of the schizophrenia and amphetamine effects do not clearly support the amphetamine model of psychosis, but the specific restriction of the effects to the N120 component, to low-intensity stimuli and to visual attention conditions suggest some commonality. The similarity of schizophrenic attentional effects (fig. 3) to figure 1 [*Buchsbaum* et al., 1978] showing attentional effects in low MAO low DBH subjects is also of neurochemical interest.

The observed differences between schizophrenics and normals do not appear attributable to either eye movements or slow negative waves. Eye movements

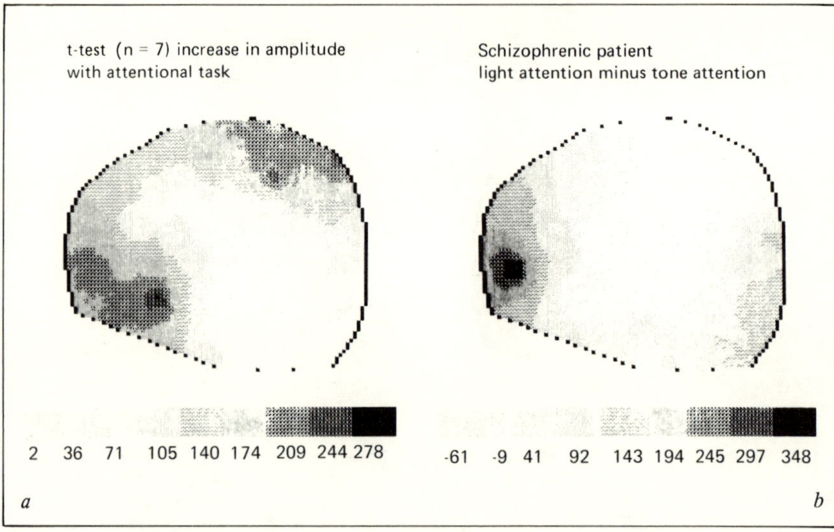

Fig. 5. ***a*** Topographic map indicating paired t-values for 7 normal subjects from comparison of visual EP N120 amplitude during attention to visual stimuli and during attention to auditory stimuli. Scale is t-value × 100. A parietal and a frontal area of significance appear. *b* Map of Attentional enhancement (calculated as in fig. 4a in a single off-medication male patient with schizophrenia. Scale is microvolts × 100. Note absence of attentional effect in parietal cortex, but continued presence in frontal cortex, and appearance of occipital pole effect not seen in figure 5.

were systematically edited out and, further, effects were maximal in parietal not frontal areas where eye movement artifacts if present, would be greatest. Digital filtering removed low frequencies below 4 Hz, thus minimizing any slow negative component contribution to the N120 attention effect. Despite filtering, the N120 attentional effect reached statistical significance with only 7 subjects.

Differences between Cz or temporoparietal cortex and Oz in visual EP attentional effects have been reported previously [*Van Voorhis and Hillyard,* 1977; *Buchsbaum and Drago,* 1977], but these studies each contained only two leads. The attention enhancement map (fig. 4, 5) suggest that we have not chosen the optimal area for schizophrenia-normal differences with the *Matsumiya* et al. [1972] W_3 area. *Shagass* et al. [1980] also showed topographic differences in N130 for somatosensory stimuli, but did not use an attentional task. Comprehensive multilead attention studies will be necessary to understand differences in the cortical patterns of attention enhancement.

Summary

The effect of selective attention on the N120 component of the visual evoked response (EP) is demonstrated in 34 normal volunteers, with an increase in temporoparietal areas after administration of amphetamine. A group of 26 off-medication schizophrenics shows less increase in N120 amplitude with selective attention. EP topographic maps of the left hemisphere based on 16 EEG leads in 7 normal volunteers confirm a parietal maximum for N120 attentional effects. The reverse of this pattern was seen in a single off-medication schizophrenic patient, the first of an ongoing series.

References

Buchsbaum, M.S.: Neurophysiological aspects of the schizophrenic syndrome; in Bellak, Disorders of the schizophrenic syndrome (Basic Books, New York 1979).

Buchsbaum, M.S.; Drago, D.: Hemispheric asymmetry in the effects of attention in the visual evoked response; in Desmedt, Language and hemispheric specialization in man: event-related cerebral potentials (Karger, Basel 1977).

Buchsbaum, M.S.; Murphy, D.L.; Coursey, R.D.; Lake, C.R.; Zeigler, M.G.: Platelet monoamine oxidase, plasma dopamine-beta-hydroxylase and attention in a 'biochemical high risk' sample. J. psychiat. Res. *14:* 215–224 (1978).

Buchsbaum, M.S.; Post, R.M.; Bunney, W.E.; Jr.: AER in a rapidly cycling manic-depressive patient. Biol. Psychiat. *12:* 83–99 (1977).

Coppola, R.: A table-driven system for stimulus-reponse experiments. Proc. Digital Equipment Users Society, Maynard 1977.

Douglas, V.I.; Virginia, I.: Higher mental processes in hyperactive children: implications for training; in Knights, Bakker, Rehabilitation, treatment, and management of learning disorders (University Park Press, Baltimore, in press).

Douglas, V.I.: Stop, look, and listen: the problems of sustained attention and impulse control in hyperactive and normal children. Can. J. Behav. Sci./Rev. Can. Sci. Comp. *4:* 259–282 (1972).

Garmezy, N.: Attentional processes in adult schizophrenia and in children at risk. J. psychiat. Res. *14:* 3–34 (1978).

Hillyard, S.A.; Picton, T.W.; Regan, D.: Sensation, perception and attention: analysis using ERPs; in Callaway, Tueting, Koslow, Event-related brain potentials in man (Academic Press, New York 1978).

Lavine, R.A.; Buchsbaum, M.S.; Schlechter, G.: Human somatosensory evoked responses: effects of attention and distraction on early components. Physiol. Psychol. *8:* 105–108 (1980).

Lehmann, D.; Skrandies, W.: Reference-free identification of components of checkerborard-evoked multichannel potential fields. Electroenceph. clin. Neurophysiol. *48:* 609–621 (1980).

Matsumiya, Y.; Tagliasco, V.; Lombroso, C.T.; Goodglass, H.: Auditory evoked response: meaningfulness of stimuli and interhemispheric asymmetry. Science *175:* 790–792 (1972).

Matthyssee, S.: Missing links; in Wynne, Cromwell, Matthyssee, The nature of schizophrenia (Wiley & Sons, New York 1978).

Meltzer, H.Y.: Biology of schizophrenia subtypes: a review and proposal for method of study. Schiz. Bull. *5:* 460–479 (1979).

Nurnberger, J.I.; Gershon, E.S.; Jimerson, D.C.; Buchsbaum, M.S.; Gold, P.; Brown, G.; Ebert, M.: Pharmacogenetics of *d*-amphetamine response in man; in Gershon, Matthysse, Breakefield, Ciaranello, Genetic research strategies for psychobiology and psychiatry (Boxwood Press, Pacific Grove 1981).

Ragot, R.A.; Remond, A.: EEG field mapping. Electroenceph. clin. Neurophysiol. *45:* 417–421 (1978).

Reuss, V.I.; Buchsbaum, M.S.; Post, R.M.: *D*-amphetamine: differential effects on right and left hemispheres, in Gruzelier, Flor-Henry, Hemisphere asymmetries of functions in psychopathology (Elsevier/North-Holland/Biomedical Press, Amsterdam 1979).

Schechter, G.; Buchsbaum, M.: The effects of attention, stimulus intensity, and individual differences on the average evoked response. Psychophysiology *10:* 392–400 (1973).

Schneider, R.D.; Grossi, V.: Differences in muscle activity before, during, and after responding in a simple reaction time task: schizophrenics vs. normals. Psychiat. Res. *1:* 141–145 (1979).

Schwent, V.L.; Snyder, E.; Hillyard, S.A.: Auditory evoked potentials during multichannel selective listening cues. J. exp. Psychol. *2:* 313–325 (1976).

Shagass, C.; Ornitz, E.M.; Sutton, S.; Tueting, P.: Event related potentials and psychopathology; in Callaway, Tueting, Koslow, Event-related potentials in man (Academic Press, New York 1978).

Shagass, C.; Roemer, R.; Straumanis, J.; Amadeo, M.: Topography of sensory evoked potentials in depressive disorders. Biol. Psychiat. *15:* 183–207 (1980).

Spitzer, R.; Endicott, J.: A diagnostic interview: The schedule for affective disorders and schizophrenia. Archs gen. Psychiat. *35:* 837–844 (1978).

Van Voorhis, S.; Hillyard, S.A.: Visual evoked potentials and selective attention to points in space. Percept. Psychophys. *22:* 54–62 (1977).

M.S. Buchsbaum, MD, Clinical Center, 2N212, Bethesda, MD 20205 (USA)

Adv. biol. Psychiat., vol. 6, pp. 195–198 (Karger, Basel 1981)

Concluding Remarks

Interaction between Neurophysiological Activities and Psychopathological Events

D. Kemali

Department of Psychiatry, 1st School of Medicine, University of Naples, Naples, Italy

To make concluding remarks to this Symposium on Clinical Neurophysiological Aspects of Psychopathological Conditions is a hard task, because of the mass of data each one of us has been acquainted with, during four intensive working sessions.

I would not run the risk of introducing confusion by comments to the contributions we have been listening to, since these comments must be pondered over as well as matched and integrated with personal knowledge and experience. Only in this way might they become useful for further progress. The alternative could be a synthesis but this would be repetitive. Therefore, I shall not attempt to produce a synthesis, but I shall take my cue from what was said, for some remarks at a more general level.

The adherence to some statements in the introductory remarks means, at the moment of closure, that we are urged by the need of an agreement on common language, both theoretical and conceptual, to be used above individual competences.

Above this and beyond this, common planning and common selection of topics to be put into focus by deeper research, as well as reciprocal validating of procedures may lead, within reasonable limits, to comparability results.

I feel that, starting from the initiative taken last year, a guideline is emerging from our work: an approach that tries to put in contact the general physiological side with the detailed pathological one, and is based on continuous methodological scrutiny. These are the criteria which have been followed here in the sequence of presentations at each session. Thus, we are becoming aware that specific conceptual contributions of experienced scientists, working in different disciplines, may determine the birth of a 'matrix disciplinaria', in the sense of the words of *Kuhn* [1970], in this area of psychiatric research.

I believe that the time has arrived for each one of us to consider our meeting not a step 'toward what we want to know' but more as an undertaking to allow us to 'start from what we know' today.

There is an implicit trap in the use of technologies, which may lead, in perspective, to mechanistic or otherwise reductionistic evaluations of results so far obtained. In my opinion, it is a lucky circumstance that available data have not produced hurried theories which, as they usually are liable not to be corroborated by further studies, frequently lack epistemic reliability.

Looking for a general framework, the basic assumptions of genetic psychology might provide a theoretical approach that could be transferred into the psychiatric field. Research should be aimed at finding possible relationships between brain *'structuring mechanisms'* and the dynamic emergence of resulting psychologically *'structured events'.*

In this view, *the adaption derives from the mutual interdependence of the assimilation of the environment into the inner biological patterns and the accommodation or tuning of these inner attributes to the external reality;* in other words, a cybernetic balance is achieved.

Furthermore, when *Piaget* [1941, 1970] stresses the relationship between nervous structures and operational psychological events, during ontological development, he proposes nothing but the concept that biological events continue into psychological ones, and that the latter, in turn, shape the biological events themselves.

This proposition may be integrated by taking into account the ideas of *Vygotskij* [1962] with which *Piaget* agreed. This is founded on the impact that cultural and social determinants have in influencing patterns of behavioral responses. In other words an anticipated recognition of a perceived stimulus is a function of the system of cognitive relational signs which mediate the direction of brain structuring mechanisms. In short, the psychological event, when it emerges from the structures, realizes and operates once again, a contact with the socio-cultural environment and consequently new dynamic structuring mechanisms.

Therefore, I am inclined to believe that, at the clinical level, we cannot consider pathology as an antagonistic state to physiology, but rather its continuation, albeit under changed conditions. Thus when, for whatever reason, we hear something which has no physical reality in the outside world, our evoked internal psychological states are just like those that could be evoked by a *real* sound. Our inner reality is just as *true* as if it were a response to an outside stimulus.

The need for defining objects of research and choosing procedures to be applied is not merely a repetition of current issues but the evidence of a frustrating experience we feel sometimes in our everyday work.

The great difficulties we are still facing may be overcome by sharpening our abilities to better define those psychological elements which result from a common mechanism that introduces detectable variations at the neurophysiological level.

Coming back to the specific interest in the correlations between brain activities and psychological events, the more attention we pay to identify related variables and their weight, the closer we should arrive to the probability of understanding the subsystem involved in the emergence of psychological features.

I hope, if we are all in agreed, that the above-mentioned theoretical framework could stimulate a fruitful convergence of multidisciplinary interests. In this case, our task should be to indicate the area of practicable approaches as well as to define validated methodologies finalizing our joint efforts towards a common goal.

'The truth may emerge from error never from confusion' [*Kuhn,* 1970]. In this perspective, I think that we should try to concentrate on circumstances that allow us to collect and interpret some indicators to which we may attribute the meaning of reliable signs.

May I be permitted a suggestion, which echoes what many of us have felt and expressed during our discussion here. I would suggest that the time is ripe for setting up a small international committee that would propose, and publicize, a minimum standard set of data that should be collected at the clinical, electrophysiological and technical levels as part of every clinical neurophysiological study on mental disease.

As a results of this, general comparisons between studies would be made possible – which they are *not* now. Furthermore, this may allow meaningful *pooling* of some data, to good advantage and, conversely, *avoid the risk* of pooling the unpoolable, with all its attendant pitfalls.

I have spoken more than I meant to. But before closing it is my sad duty to commemorate with you *Piaget.* I could not do better than to do so by quoting from his *Réussir et comprendre* [1974] in which he attempts an analysis of what are the features in common as well as the differences between, on the one hand, the states of 'achieving a result', which implies 'knowing what to do' and, on the other hand, the states of 'understanding', which characterizes conceptualization.

The latter is characterized by the fact that while understanding may well be the result of a given series of actions, above all it can proceed and indeed direct action itself. We may conclude, with *Piaget* [1974], that when we resolve some research issues, most others remain unresolved and, though this may produce disquiet in some, it may not be so for the researcher who finds the new questions even more previous than the achieved solutions.

Concluding our meeting, I wish to express again my thanks to all the speakers who have offered us the possibility of sharing their knowledge, the participants for their stimulating contributions and my colleagues and friends *L. Vacca, A. Amati,* and *M. Del Vecchio,* for their help.

Let me express my warmest thanks to Prof. *P.E. Polani,* for his sharp criticism and his friendly help have made clear my own thought, giving a further evidence of interdisciplinary impact.

Thank you all again.

References

Kuhn, T.S.: The structure of scientific revolutions. (University of Chicago Press, Chicago 1970).

Piaget, J.: Le mécanisme du dévoloppement mental et les lois du groupement des opérations. Esquisse d'une théorie opératoire de l'intelligence. Archs Psychol. *28:* 215–285 (1941).

Piaget, J.: La situation des sciences de l'homme dans le système des sciences; tendences principales de la rechèrche deans les sciences sociales et humaines. Prémière partie: sciences sociales (Montore, Le Hague UNESCO, Paris 1970).

Piaget, J.: Réussir et comprendre (Presses universitaires de France, Paris 1974).

Vygotskij, L.S.: in Hanfmann, Vakar, Thought and language (MIT Press, Chicago 1962).

D. Kemali, MD, Institute of Psychiatry, First Medical School, University of Naples, I-80100 Naples (Italy).

Subject Index